Breast Cancer and its Precursor Lesions

CURRENT CLINICAL PATHOLOGY

ANTONIO GIORDANO, MD, PHD

SERIES EDITOR

For other titles published in this series, go to
www.springer.com/series/7632

Patricia A. Thomas

Editor

Breast Cancer
and its Precursor Lesions

Making Sense and Making It Early

✻ Humana Press

Editor
Patricia A. Thomas
Professor of Pathology and Surgery
University of Kansas Medical Center
Office of Cultural Enhancement and Diversity
Kansas City, KS
USA
pthomas@kumc.edu

ISBN 978-1-58829-686-3   e-ISBN 978-1-60327-154-7
DOI 10.1007/978-1-60327-154-7
Springer New York Dordrecht Heidelberg London

Library of Congress Control Number: 2010937418

Humana Press is part of Springer Science+Business Media (www.springer.com)

Preface

Pathologists are physicians who play a critical role in the diagnosis and management of disease. The responsibility of the pathologist in evaluating abnormalities of the breast is to establish accurate, thorough, and timely diagnoses by carefully examining the tissue and cells that are comprising a given abnormality. The pathologist generates a report to communicate their diagnoses and impressions, but sometimes that report can be not readily and unequivocally interpreted by non-pathologists. It has been reported that surgeons misunderstood pathology reports 30% of the time. For patients, the diagnoses that pathologists make can be life altering, so the pathology report and a clear understanding of that report should be particularly important to these stakeholders. And, if it wasn't a challenge already for non-pathologists to interpret and understand the pathology report, increased appreciation of the range of types and behaviors of cancerous and precancerous breast diseases and advances in knowledge and techniques available for pathologic evaluation of tissue and cells have led to increasingly complex reports.

This book will cover the common breast conditions and diseases, using contemporary terminology and accompanying illustrations. Our aim is to create a book that will help other clinicians, residents, and even patients "decipher" the language of breast pathology and better understand the pathology report.

Kansas City, KS   Patricia A. Thomas

Contents

Contributors

Joan Cangiarella, MD
Associate Professor, Department of Pathology,
New York University School of Medicine, New York, NY, USA
joan.cangiarella@nymc.org

Fang Fan, MD/PhD
Associate Professor, Department of Pathology and Laboratory Medicine,
University of Kansas Medical Center, Kansas City, KS, USA
ffan@kumc.edu

Patricia A. Thomas, MD/MA/FCAP/FASCP
Professor, Department of Pathology and Laboratory Medicine,
University of Kansas Medical Center, Kansas City, KS, USA
pthomas@kumc.edu

Chapter 1
Overview

Patricia A. Thomas

Keywords Incidence • Epidemiology • Risk factors • Mutation • Basal type • Geography • Health disparities • Access to care • Estrogen exposure • Pathology report • Predictive markers • Prognostic markers • Race/ethnicity • Culture • Molecular profiling • Genetic profiling

Introduction

Breast cancer has been described in written records for millennia; it knows no racial/ethnic, socioeconomic, health, regal, celebrity, political, cultural, geographic, or temporal boundaries [1]. The breast has been depicted in some of our most treasured and ancient art and literature. For the ancients, "breast cancer was cancer" [1]. Other cancers surely existed but those were not readily seen or appreciated. As the purpose of the breast is production of milk for the nourishment of infants or small children, the breast can be viewed as symbolic of motherhood and being female, and for many emblematic of sexuality. These symbolic associations have been depicted in art and literature across the ages [1]. Thus the cultural and personal aspects of a breast cancer diagnosis are important considerations. There is no doubt that these two factors, in addition to ever expanding medical/scientific knowledge and technical advances, have influenced our concepts about breast cancer behavior and treatment over time.

P.A. Thomas (✉)
Professor, Department of Pathology and Laboratory Medicine, University of Kansas Medical Center, Kansas City, KS, USA
e-mail: pthomas@kumc.edu

P.A. Thomas (ed.), *Breast Cancer and its Precursor Lesions*, Current Clinical Pathology, DOI 10.1007/978-1-60327-154-7_1, © Springer Science+Business Media, LLC 2011

Incidence and Epidemiology

Breast cancer is currently the most common cancer (excluding skin cancers) in woman. It is second only to lung cancer as a cause of cancer-related deaths in woman. More than 192,000 women were diagnosed with invasive breast cancer in 2009 and more than 40,000 women died from this disease [2]. One in eight women who lives upto 90 years of age will be diagnosed with cancer [3]. There are over 2.5 million breast cancer survivors in the USA [2].

With the advent of screening mammography in the early 1980s there was increase in the incidence (occurrence) of breast cancer. This trend continued over many years, until breast cancer incidence started to decline in 1999 [2, 3]. Breast cancer-related deaths have also been declining since the 1990s [2, 3]. Increased patient education and awareness regarding screening mammography, breast self examination and the clinical breast examination, advances in imaging, adherence to screening recommendations, and improved therapies in combination account for that decline. However, the decline for African American and other non-European American women has not been as great [3]. Nonetheless, the decrease in the numbers of new breast cancers holds promise.

Risk Factors

Among the risk factors or determinants (conditions) associated with breast cancer, gender is the most important; male breast cancer accounts for only 1% of all breast cancer cases [2, 3]. Besides hereditary breast cancers, and those cancers related to early radiation exposure, the major risk factors are linked to duration of estrogen exposure: gender, age at first menstrual cycle (less than 12 years of age), age at menopause (greater than 55 years of age), age at birth of first child (30 years old or more), not having children, breastfeeding and exogenous (introduced and produced outside the body) hormones [2, 3]. It is hypothesized that the cycles of cellular proliferation stimulated by estrogen increases the opportunities for proliferating cells to undergo permanent DNA damage or mutation. As the mutations accumulate, abnormal cells are generated that are no longer controlled by normal cellular control programs and cancer develops.

Some risk factors are beyond the control of patients; others are modifiable life-style choices. See Table 1.1. Women who have full-term pregnancies at 20 years of age and younger have about half the risk of developing breast cancer as women who never have children or women who have their first full-term baby after the age of 30 years [3]. The reasons for these observations are, as previously mentioned related to estrogen exposure, i.e., fewer menstrual cycles, decreasing the opportunities for DNA damage and mutation, which are necessary steps in the development of non-hereditary breast cancer. During lactation there would be fewer menstrual cycles as well. Another hypothesis about pregnancy and lactation is that a full-term pregnancy results in terminal or completion of differentiation of milk-producing

Table 1.1 Breast cancer risk factors

Risk factors: unchangeable	Risk factors: changeable
Gender	No children or later age at first live birth
Age	No breastfeeding
Genetics (hereditary breast cancers)	Hormone replacement treatment
Family history (first degree relative) or personal history	Birth control pills (recent use)
Race/ethnicity	Geography
Dense breast tissue	Alcohol (moderate consumption)
Younger age at onset of menstrual periods/later age at onset of menopause	Post-menopausal obesity
Radiation to chest early in life	Lack of exercise

cells which decreases the potential pool of mutated cells or cancer precursors. For women over 30 years of age it is thought that this protective effect is outweighed by the number of cells that have already undergone precancerous changes and the abnormal cells are stimulated in early pregnancy [3]. For African American women, however, age at first full-term birth is not a strong risk factor [3].

Estrogen exposure in the form of hormone replacement therapy slightly increases the risk of breast cancer [2, 3]. Some studies suggest that women who use oral contraceptives have a slightly increased risk over women who have never used them; however, that risk goes back to normal as soon as a woman stops taking them [2]. The increased risk in post-menopausal obese patients is likely related to the estrogens being produced in fatty tissue [3]. Exercise appears to have a protective effect that is greatest for premenopausal women, women who have had full-term pregnancies and for women who are not obese [3]. Geography plays an interesting role in breast cancer with breast cancer incidence rates being four to seven times higher in the USA and Europe than incidence rates in other countries [3]. For women who immigrate to the USA from a country with a low incidence of breast cancer, the risk of breast cancer increases with each successive generation [3]. Associations between breast cancer rates, geographic location, and level of sun exposure have been described, with higher rates of breast cancer in countries at latitudes further away from the equator [4] and/or decreased sun exposure [5] and suggest a protective effect for vitamin D.

Race/Ethnicity and Culture

Racial/ethnic differences in breast cancer are examples of the many health disparities that exist in the USA [6–8]. Disparities in the breast cancer experience and outcomes across racial/ethnic lines are serious issues. Many researchers have focused their on understanding the basis of these differences and eventually eliminating such health disparities [6]. Breast cancer occurs less often in African American, Hispanic/Latino, and Native American patients than in women of European ancestry when viewed across all age groups; but, these women often present with advanced or higher stage (burden of disease or how widespread) disease. African American women have the highest rates of death from breast cancer, followed by non-Hispanic whites and trailed by Hispanic, Native American, Alaska Native, Asian and Pacific Islander women [6, 7]. Native American and Alaska Natives have lowest incidence [6, 7]. However, when Native American women are diagnosed with cancers, the outcomes are poor [6]. The reasons for these differences are multifactorial.

While access to care is an issue and health insurance is but one aspect of access, studies have shown that racial differences in the breast cancer experience persist when access and other clinical, demographic and socioeconomic factors were controlled [6]. African American women are less likely to receive standard of care or equal treatment compared to their white counterparts [6]. In addition, there is growing evidence the biology may account for some racial disparities in breast cancer [1, 9]. African American woman are more likely to have highly aggressive tumors with unfavorable prognostic (a forecast of the likely course and outcome of disease) factors [6]. Genetic studies have shown that breast cancers in African American women, especially premenopausal, are likely to be of the basal-type, which is a very aggressive form of the disease [10]. In fact, among women under 30 years of age African Americans have a higher rate of breast cancer compared to whites [11]. The converse is true overall, as stated above, but especially after age 40 years [11].

The symbolic associations of motherhood, being female, and sexuality associated with breasts would suggest that there are important cultural and personal factors to consider. No doubt cultural and personal influences have influenced how we treat and think about breast cancer over time. Cultural and personal differences in attitudes, beliefs, and practices vary across groups and in part contribute to racial/ethnic differences seen in breast cancer [12]. There are some African Americans that believe the "devil" causes cancer or that breast surgery will make them no longer attractive to men [12]. In the Navajo language the literal translation for cancer is "the sore that never heals," leading some Native American women to believe that a breast cancer diagnosis is a death decree for which there is no help [7, 13]. Native Americans and Alaskan may view cancer as a punishment and may not discuss it for fear of stigma and shame [7, 13]. Health-related beliefs and behaviors vary across groups and are important factors to consider. These differences in attitudes, beliefs, and behaviors are obviously not limited to patients and these differences influence physician behaviors at time as illustrated by the unequal treatment African American experience [6].

Prognostic and Predictive Factors

A prognostic factor, as mentioned above, is one that forecasts the likely course of or outcome of disease, i.e., the likelihood of cure or not. A predictive factor is one that provides information that predicts whether a given tumor will respond to a given therapy. These factors included characteristics of the tumor, such as size, type, stage (extent of disease or how wide spread), grade (how closely the tumor cells resemble the cell of origin), and cellular proteins or genes involved in breast cancer. Advances in technology and knowledge about breast cancer have resulted in an increase in the number of these factors available to evaluate. Some are still being studied to determine their true usefulness in providing reliable prognostic and/or predictive information. Type of tumor, grade, and stage remain the most powerful prognostic features to date. Hormone receptor status (receptor protein present), and the epidermal growth factor B2 receptor known as Her-2/neu stand apart, so far, as strong predictive factors. Molecular and genetic profiling results are promising as well.

The role of the pathologist in breast cancer diagnosis is rarely directly discussed; however, treatment and management decisions rely upon the pathologist's accurate, thorough, and timely diagnosis. The pathology report that is generated is a very important part of the patient's medical record, as it drives treatment and management decision for breast cancer patients. This report contains the diagnosis, information necessary to determine extent of disease and biological potential of the cancer, forecast the probable course or outcome for the patient, establish that the cancer is completely removed, and assist other doctors in determining choice of therapy and predicting the effectiveness of a particular therapy. The increasing practice of breast conservation, neoadjuvant chemotherapy, and novel prognostic and predictive factors have added necessary complexity to pathology reports.

An unequivocal understanding of the pathology report is important and the responsibility of communicating the information in the pathology report is that of the treating physician. However, it has been reported that surgeons misunderstood pathology reports 30% of the time [14]. Experienced surgeons were less likely to interpret reports erroneously [14]. It is therefore important that the surgeon, oncologist, or radiation oncologist seek clarification from the pathologist and even review the report in detail with the pathologist. Consultation, collaboration and active participation as a member of multidisciplinary team caring for breast cancer patients are arguably the pathologist's most important roles. Finding, diagnosing, and treating breast cancer at an early stage positively impacts survival. Misunderstandings of the pathology report should not play any part in delay of or suboptimal care.

For the most part, the pathologist who produces the pathology report does not have direct patient contact. In fact, pathologists in fact are often referred to or refer to themselves as the "doctor's doctor". However, given the life-altering nature of a cancer diagnosis for patients and their families, the extent and increasing complexity of a breast cancer pathology report and the increased involvement of women in their own care, it would not be unreasonable for those patients inclined to do so to seek information about their reports directly from the pathologist. The pathology report could be used as a powerful educational tool for the patient who has been diagnosed with breast cancer [15].

In this book, we will discuss some of the common breast conditions, cancer precursors, cancers, nuances of diagnosing breast cancer, and how to read the pathology report using contemporary terminology in easy to understand language and accompanying illustrations. Our aim is to create a book that will help other clinicians, residents, and even patients "decipher" the language of breast pathology and better understand the pathology report.

References

1. Olson J (2002) Dark ages. Bathsheba's breast: women, cancer and history, 1st edn. John Hopkins University Press, Baltimore, MD
2. Overview: Breast Cancer (2009) http://www.cancer.org/docroot/CRI/CRI_2_1x. asp?rnav=criov&dt=5 Accessed 12 Dec 2009
3. Lester SC (2008) The breast. In: Kumar V, Abbas A , Fausto, N, and Aster, JC. (eds) Robins and Cotran Pathologic basis of disease, 8th edn. Saunders, Philadelphia, pp 1065–1071
4. Mohr SB, Garland CF, Gorham ED, Grant WB, Garland FC (2008) Relationship between low ultraviolet B irradiance and higher breast cancer risk in 107 countries. Breast J 14(3):255–260
5. Millen AE, Pettinger M, Freudenheim JL, Langer RD, Rosenberg CA, Mossavar-Rahmani Y, Duffy CM, Lane DS, McTiernan A, Kuller LH, Lopez AM, Wactawski-Wende J (2009) Incident invasive breast cancer, geographic location of residence, and reported average time spent outside. Cancer Epidemiol Biomarkers Prev 18(2):495–507
6. Institute of Medicine of the National Academies (2003) Introduction and literature review. In: Smedley BD, Smith AY, Nelson AR (eds) Unequal treatment: confronting racial and ethnic disparities in health care. National Academies, Washington, DC, pp 52–57
7. Leigh WA, Huff D (2006) Women of color health data book: adolescents to seniors. National Institute of Health, Washington
8. Fiscella K; Franks P; Gold MR; Clancy CM (2000) Inequality in quality: addressing socio-economic, racial, and ethnic disparities in health care. JAMA 283:2579–2584
9. Amend K, Hicks D, Ambrosone CB (2006) Breast cancer in African-American Women: differences in tumor biology from European-American women. Cancer Res 66:8327–8330
10. Klauber-DeMore N (2005–2006) Tumor biology of breast cancer in young women. Breast Dis 23:9–15
11. Brinton LA, Sherman ME, Carreon JD, Anderson WF (2008) Recent trends in breast cancer among younger women in the United States. J Natl Cancer Inst 100(22):1643–1648
12. Lannin DR, Mathews HF, Mitchell J, Swanson MS, Swanson FH, Edwards MS (1998) Influence of socioeconomic and cultural factors on racial differences in late-stage presentation of breast cancer. JAMA 279:1801–1807
13. Robinson F, Sandoval N, Baldwin J, Sanderson PR (2005) Breast cancer education for native American women: creating culturally relevant communications. Clin J Oncol Nurs 9(6):689–692
14. Powsner S, Costa J, Homer R (2002) Clinicians are from mars and pathologists are from venus. Clinician interpretations of pathology reports. Arch Pathol Lab Med 124:1040–1046
15. Strobel SL, Tatchell T (2002) The surgical pathology report as an educational tool for cancer patients. Ann Clin Lab Sci 32:363–368

Chapter 2
Common Benign Conditions of Low Concern

Fang Fan and Patricia A. Thomas

Keywords Anatomy • Terminal duct lobular unit (f) • Luminal cells • Myoepithelial cells • Acinus (f) • Basement membrane • Lactation • Benign conditions • Reactive conditions • Inflammatory conditions • Acute mastitis (f) • Subareolar abscess (f) • Mammary duct ectasia (f) • Fat necrosis (f) • Lymphocytic mastopathy (f) • Diabetic mastopathy (f) • Nonproliferative fibrocystic changes

It is necessary to give a brief overview of the structure of the breast in order to put into context the various conditions that will be described in this chapter and others. The breast is comprised of fat, connective tissue, and glands (ducts and lobules) (see Fig. 2.1a). The amount of connective tissue also called stroma varies among women. When it is increased it leads to a denser breast, it may make the detection of cancer by mammography more difficult. The ratio of fatty tissue to glandular tissue varies among women and at different times in woman's life. In younger woman the ratio usually favors the glandular tissue. After menopause as the number of glands diminishes, the ratio favors the fatty. Weight gain or loss affects this ratio as well. The majority of a woman's glandular tissue is situated near the axilla or under arm, in the upper outer quadrant (about 10 o'clock if you were to imagine the breast with a clock superimposed) where a majority of cancers occur.

To understand the majority of conditions that arise in the breast, we will focus on the anatomy of glands (lobules and ducts), which are formed by epithelium. Epithelium is the layer of tissue that covers the outer part of the body and lines those inner surfaces of the body that communicate with or have some connection to the outside world.

The breast contains six to ten major ducts which branch into smaller ducts that eventually connect to the terminal ductal lobular unit [1]. The terminal ducts branch into clusters of acini (more than one acinus) (see Fig. 2.1b). These grape-like clusters form the lobules of the breast. Two cell types comprise the epithelium

F. Fan (✉)
Associate Professor, Department of Pathology and Laboratory Medicine,
University of Kansas Medical Center, Kansas City, KS, USA
e-mail: ffan@kumc.edu

P.A. Thomas (ed.), *Breast Cancer and its Precursor Lesions*, Current Clinical Pathology,
DOI 10.1007/978-1-60327-154-7_2, © Springer Science+Business Media, LLC 2011

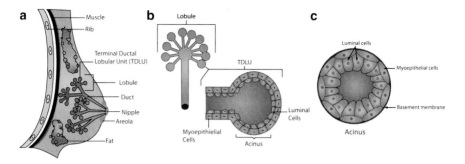

Fig. 2.1 Schematic drawings of a cross-section of breast, the terminal ductal lobular unit and acinus. (**a**) Depicts a cross-section of the breast and its contents. (**b**) Illustrates the terminal ductal lobular unit and its relationship to the lobule. The circular projections of the terminal ductal lobular unit are representations of the acini that also comprise the lobule. (**c**) Illustrates the details of a single acinus.

that lines the ducts and lobules (see Fig. 2.1b). The bottom layer of cells are myoepithelial cells, which stretch out in a mesh-like fashion along what is called the basement membrane, the supporting layer of tissue that separates the epithelium from the tissue beneath it. Myoepithelial cells have contractile properties and assist with milk ejection during lactation and provide support for the lobules. Luminal epithelial cells (usually cube-like or cuboidal in shape) sit vertically above the myoepithelial cells (see Fig. 2.1c). Normally the cells that comprise the epithelial layer are attached to each other and the basement membrane tightly enough to form a continuous protective barrier, a property that is disrupted in cancer. See Fig. 2.1c which shows an acinus and the two cell layer arrangement.

The terminal ductal lobular unit is the functional unit of the breast. The luminal epithelial cells that line the acini produce and secrete milk during lactation. The breast is never fully differentiated or mature until a woman carries a birth to term and lactates, which is significant because full maturation is protective against breast cancer. The terminal ductal lobular unit is also where it is believed that all precancerous and cancers lesions arise, the majority of which are epithelial [2].

This overview of breast anatomy should provide a better understanding of the various conditions that will be discussed.

Benign Conditions Associated with No Risk

Benign breast conditions represent a spectrum of changes that may be associated with breast pain, lumpiness, a well-defined mass that can be felt, and nipple discharge. Most breast abnormalities are benign; however, biopsy may be required to distinguish some of these benign abnormalities from malignancy. Benign breast abnormalities are generally divided into two categories based on their association with breast cancer: one group has no increased risk for developing breast cancer and the other group has an increased risk of developing breast cancer. This chapter describes the first group of benign abnormalities that have no increased risk of developing breast cancer as compared to women in general population who do not have biopsy proven abnormalities.

Reactive and inflammatory lesions

Acute mastitis almost always occurs when a woman's breast is producing milk (lactation period) and presents as unilateral, erythematous, and painful mass. Biopsies from this condition are uncommon. By microscope the tissue shows collections of inflammatory cells (neutrophils) and ductal epithelium that may show reactive changes because of the inflammation. This condition is treated by antibiotics and complete drainage of milk.

Subareolar abscess has a strong association with cigarette smoking. Clinical presentations include painful erythematous subareolar mass and abnormal mammograms. This lesion is associated with squamous metaplasia of large or lactiferous ducts, subsequent formation of keratin plug, rupture, and inflammatory response [1]. Fine needle aspiration shows anucleated keratin debris associated with inflammatory cells.

Mammary duct ectasia occurs in older women and is not associated with smoking. The characteristic clinical presentation is poorly defined periareolar mass, thick-cheesy nipple discharge (tooth paste-like), and occasionally abnormal mammograms. It is usually due to inspissation of breast secretions leading to dilatation and rupture of ducts and strong inflammatory response [3]. Histology shows dilated ducts filled with foamy macrophages and surrounded by chronic inflammation and fibrosis (Fig. 2.2).

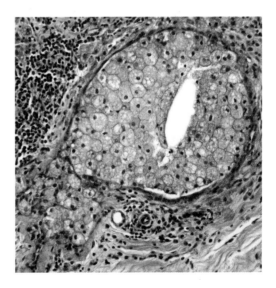

Fig. 2.2 Mammary duct ectasia. An ectatic duct is shown filled with foamy macrophages and surrounded by chronic inflammation and fibrosis.

Fig. 2.3 Fat necrosis. There are dilated spaces surrounded by lipid-laden foamy macrophages and foreign body giant cells.

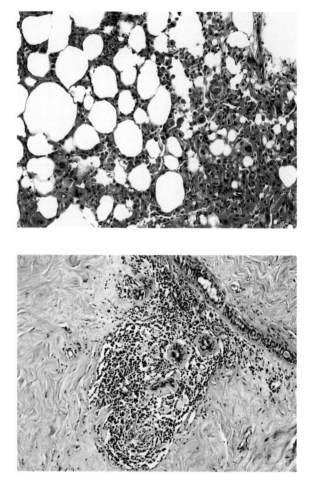

Fig. 2.4 Diabetic mastopathy. The biopsy specimen shows keloid-like stroma fibrosis and lobular lymphocytic infiltrates.

Fat necrosis of the breast usually follows a prior history of trauma or surgery; however, in many cases, a history of injury may not be elicited. It may present clinically as a palpable mass or mammographic calcifications concerning for malignancy. Histologically, it shows variable cystic spaces representing necrotic fat cells surrounded by foamy macrophages and foreign-body type giant cells (Fig. 2.3). Sometimes, the lipid-laden foamy macrophages raise concern for carcinoma cells. Immunohistochemical stains (microscopic localization of specific markers using antibodies with dyes or enzymes that produce a color that can be visualized) for epithelial marker and histiocytic marker will help in making the correct diagnosis.

Lymphocytic mastopathy/diabetic mastopathy primarily affects women of young to middle-ages. It is commonly associated with type I diabetes. Clinically it presents as multiple or bilateral firm masses [4]. The characteristic histologic features include dense keloid-like fibrosis, lymphocytic infiltrates around ducts, within lobules and around vessels (Fig. 2.4). Complete excision is the choice of therapy although the lesion may recur even with complete excision.

Nonproliferative fibrocystic changes

Fibrocystic changes of the breast are the single most common groups of disorders of the breast for women between ages 20 and 40. Typically a young woman will have "lumpy bumpy" breasts on clinical examination. Mammogram may show a dense breast with abnormal calcifications. The term "nonproliferative" implies that significant hyperplasia of ductal epithelium is not present; therefore, this lesion confers no increased risk of developing breast carcinoma [5]. Characteristic histological features of fibrocystic changes include cysts, apocrine metaplasia of ductal epithelium, expansion of lobules (adenosis) and stromal fibrosis (Fig. 2.5). The cause of fibrocystic changes is not entirely clear and is thought to be related to a localized imbalance between estrogen and progesterone. The cysts may be visible to the unaided eye ("blue-dome" cysts), and are lined by flattened epithelium or apocrine epithelium. Cyst contents and secretory debris may calcify and be detected by mammogram. The rupture of cysts results in chronic inflammation and fibrosis of surrounding tissue. Calcifications may be present in expanded lobules or adenosis. Fibrocystic changes are not associated with an increased risk of breast cancer if the epithelium of the ducts/acini is not involved by significant epithelial hyperplasia.

Deciphering the Pathology Report

When interpreting a pathology report, it is important to know that the term "lesion" may be used to describe the structural abnormality that the radiologist has seen on imaging and the pathologist sees by microscope.

The report will also mention the method used to sample abnormalities. The above discussed benign breast entities may be seen on core needle biopsy, lumpectomy, or mastectomy specimens. On rare occasion, especially if the biopsy is small, the

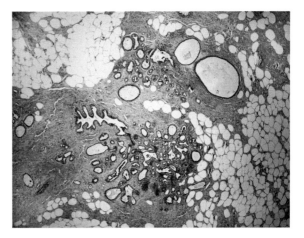

Fig. 2.5 Fibrocystic changes. Characteristic histologic features of fibrocystic changes are shown here, including cysts formation, apocrine metaplasia, and stromal fibrosis.

Fig. 2.6 Microcalcifications in benign breast lesions. Microcalcifications are identified in the cyst contents and associated with benign epithelium (arrows).

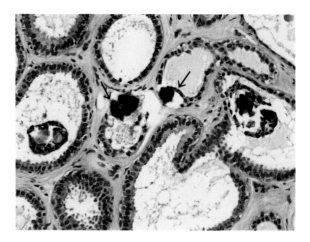

pathologist may use the term "consistent with" in the diagnosis, since all the features that are usually seen in a given abnormality, may not be present on a small biopsy.

Microcalcifications may be associated with benign breast lesions as described as above, proliferative breast lesions (Chap. 3), ductal carcinoma in situ (Chap. 4), or invasive cancers (Chap. 5). Biopsy specimens that arrive at the laboratory labeled "with microcalcifications," require pathologists have to identify microcalcifications under the microscope. The appearance and amount of microcalcifications seen by the pathologist should correlate with the microcalcifications on the mammogram that has been targeted by radiologists as the abnormality of concern. If the pathology report states that the microcalcifications are identified and associated with nonproliferative fibrocystic changes (Fig. 2.6) or any of the above lesions, then no further clinical management is needed. The report will not usually quantify the microcalcifications or mention the mammographic appearance; however, pathologists and radiologists understand the importance of pathologic and radiologic correlation and usually discuss their findings with each other.

References

1. Lester SC (2009) The breast. In: Kumar V, Abbas A, Fausto N, Aster J (eds) Pathologic basis of disease, 8th edn. Philadelphia, Saunders, pp 1069–1070
2. Wellings SR (1980) A hypothesis of the origin of human breast cancer form the terminal ductal lobular unit. Pathol Res Pract 166:515–535
3. Dixon JM, Ravisekar O, Chetty U et al (1996) Periductal mastitis and duct ectasia: different conditions with different aetiologies. Br J Surg 83:820–822
4. Ely KA, Tse G, Simpson JF et al (2000) Diabetic mastopathy. A clinicopathologic review. Am J Clin Pathol 113:541–545
5. Hartmann LC, Sellers TA, Frost MH et al (2005) Benign breast disease and the risk of breast cancer. N Engl J Med 353:229–237

Chapter 3
Benign Conditions Associated with a Risk for the Subsequent Development of Cancer

Patricia A. Thomas

Keywords Fibrocystic changes • Proliferative breast disease without atypia • Proliferative breast disease with atypia • Usual ductal hyperplasia (f) • Sclerosing adenosis (f) • Complex sclerosing lesion (f) • Marker lesions • Radial scar (f) • Papilloma (f) • Papillomatosis (f) • Relative risk • Flat epithelial lesion (f) • Upgrading • Core needle biopsy • Triple test • Chemoprevention • Estrogen receptor modulators • Columnar cell lesions • Atypical lobular hyperplasia • Lobular neoplasia • Clonal • Pagetoid

The vast majority of breast conditions that are biopsied (sampled) are benign [1]. Some of these benign conditions are associated with the increased risk for the subsequent development of cancer and some are not 1–5 Those that are associated with an elevated risk can be placed into a spectrum of changes referred to as proliferative breast disease (with or without atypia). They are considered marker lesions in contrast to precursor lesions, which will be described in Chap. 4. Marker lesions are associated with risk for cancers in both breasts. If cancer develops in the same breast as a marker lesion, it is likely to arise at a location in that breast other than where the marker lesion was found, in contrast to precursor lesions, for which subsequent cancers are usually found in close proximity to where the precursor lesion was located.

Symptoms may include breast tenderness or pain, lumpiness, irregular nodularity or well-defined mass [1]. However, most commonly these benign conditions are incidental findings in biopsies for asymptomatic mammographic findings found on screening mammography. Wide spread screening mammography has resulted in increased detection of in situ and invasive cancers, as well as these more subtle benign lesions that are associated with variable risk for the subsequent development of cancer [5, 6]. These proliferative lesions are often found adjacent to or associated with cancers on excisional biopsy or lumpectomy, therefore finding proliferative lesions on core needle biopsy specimens presents unique issues (Table 3.1).

P.A. Thomas (✉)
Professor, Department of Pathology and Laboratory Medicine, University of Kansas Medical Center, Kansas City, KS, USA
e-mail: pthomas@kumc.edu

P.A. Thomas (ed.), *Breast Cancer and its Precursor Lesions*, Current Clinical Pathology, DOI 10.1007/978-1-60327-154-7_3, © Springer Science+Business Media, LLC 2011

Table 3.1 Benign breast lesions and the relative risks associated for developing breast cancer

Nonproliferative changes – relative risk = 1.0
Cysts
Apocrine metaplasia
Duct ectasia
Non-sclerosing adenosis or sclerosing adenosis that is not florid
Mild usual ductal hyperplasia
Proliferative breast disease without atypia – relative risk = 1.5–2.0
Moderate and florid usual ductal hyperplasia
Papilloma, solitary or multiple
Florid sclerosing adenosis
Proliferative breast disease with atypia – relative risk = 4.0–5.0
Atypical ductal hyperplasia
Atypical lobular hyperplasia
Remains to be determine
Flat epithelial atypia

Proliferative breast disease diagnosed on excisional biopsy usually requires no additional surgery. A diagnosis made by needle core biopsy, may require excision [7]. Patients diagnosed with proliferative breast disease by any means do require careful follow-up. The initial risk is further increased for patients with a strong family or personal history. Such patients may choose chemoprevention using tamoxifen or other selective estrogen receptor modulators (SERMS). One large study found that the risk is also further increased when atypia is diagnosed before 45 years of age [5]. This same study reports that increased risk persists for at least 25 years after the initial biopsy [5].

Proliferative Breast Disease Without Atypia

Usual Ductal Hyperplasia

Usual ductal hyperplasia is a component of fibrocystic changes. As previously described, ducts are normally lined by two layers of cells – luminal epithelial cells and basal myoepithelial cells. An increase or proliferation in the number of luminal cells within a ductal space is considered as usual ductal hyperplasia [7,8]. The degree of proliferation or increase in number of luminal cells is varied and can range from mild (3–4 cell layers) to florid, proliferations that may fill the ductal space, see Fig. 3.1. Usual ductal hyperplasia is characterized by a heterogeneous proliferation of luminal and myoepithelial cells. Mild hyperplasia, a proliferation resulting in 3 to 4 layers, does not impart an increased risk. Moderate to florid hyperplasia, distends the lumen by a proliferation more than four cells thick and can fill and nearly obliterate the lumen is associated with a slightly increased risk. Epithelial bridges can be seen, but they are thin and tapered, with the cells unevenly distributed, see Table 3.2. These more cellular hyperplasias, in addition to filling and sometimes dilating the ductal space, feature slit like spaces; sometimes, the cells are slanted in relationship to the basement membrane and may take on a whirling or swirling pattern, see Fig. 3.1. Usual ductal hyperplasia is most frequently an incidental finding. It can be observed at any age, but the majority of women are between 35 and 60 years of age. Usual ductal hyperplasia without atypia has no widely accepted lobular counterpart. Some of the genetic alterations that are necessary for the progression to cancer have already taken place in these lesions [8].

Fig. 3.1 (**a**) Shows florid usual intraductal hyperplasia with irregularly shaped and sized spaces. (**b**) Illustrates the thin bridges, "streaming" and unevenly distributed cells.

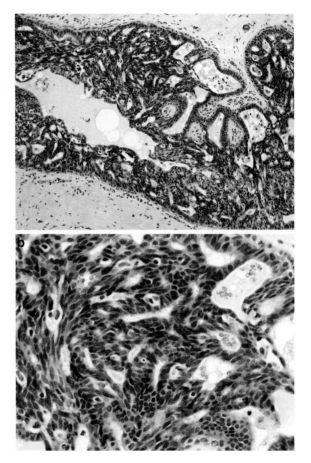

Table 3.2 Lesions diagnosed by core needle biopsy (CNB) that are associated with upgrading of the diagnosis on excision[a]

Flat epithelial atypia
Atypical ductal hyperplasia
Number of atypical epithelial foci (>2)
Presence of micropapillary architecture
Microcalcifications (when compared to masses)
Ductal carcinoma in situ
Lobular carcinoma in situ involving >50% of the CNB
Incomplete removal of the lesion

[a]Adapted from Ref. [9]

Deciphering the Pathology Report

In most cases, the pathology report should be straightforward, but there are a few things to consider. Sometimes pathology reports contain a "laundry list" of findings usually consistent with benign non-proliferative and no risk fibrocystic changes. What is important is to understand that the degree of hyperplasia varies and the term hyperplasia by itself, if present in a report, may not necessarily be referring to a lesion associated with increased risk. For example, mild hyperplasia is not associated with the subsequent risk for cancer, so the pathology report should in some way impart the degree and significance of the intraductal proliferation by indicating the degree of proliferation, i.e. mild, moderate or florid. An unqualified "hyperplasia" most likely is referring to a mild degree of proliferation. Some pathologists may distinguish mild hyperplasia and other non-proliferative conditions from the next level of proliferation, i.e. moderate to florid, by using the term proliferative breast disease without atypia to signify a proliferation that is more significant than mild hyperplasia and associated with a slightly increased risk. Others may simply use the terms moderate and/or florid usual ductal hyperplasia for the same degree of proliferation. If the reason for the biopsy was microcalcifications, the presence or absence of microcalcifications should be mentioned. In some instances, the mammographic image of the microcalcifications is sent to the laboratory for correlation with the tissue sections that are evaluated by the pathologist. It is important that the size, number and pattern are consistent with the pathology findings, regardless of whether the mammograph accompanies the specimen or not. This has been accomplished by developing effective communication and collaboration between the pathologist and radiologist.

Patients require no further treatment, but awareness that this lesion imparts a slightly increased risk for developing cancer might be important information for the patient, especially for patients with a strong family history of breast cancer.

Sclerosing Adenosis

This lobular based lesion is characterized by a disordered proliferation of epithelium, myoepithelium, and stroma. The acini are compressed centrally and increased to at least double the number in uninvolved lobules. Acini on the periphery may remain open, see Fig. 3.2. The lobule maintains its lobular organization, but is enlarged and distorted by the proliferating fibrous tissue. Sclerosing adenosis may present as a mass or a suspicious mammographic finding, or be an incidental finding. It can sometimes be associated with symptoms of pain and tenderness of the breast. Sclerosis adenosis is often associated with other proliferative lesions, such as usual ductal hyperplasia, papillomas, and complex sclerosing lesions (radial scars). Microcalcifications may be present. In fact, in order of frequency, the five most common lesions associated with microcalcifications are: fibrocystic changes, fibroadenomas, ductal carcinoma in situ, sclerosing adenosis, and columnar cell

Fig. 3.2 Illustrates the heterogenous proliferation of sclerosing adenosis, with increased and compact acini, fibrosis or sclerosis, compressed acini centrally and open acini peripherally.

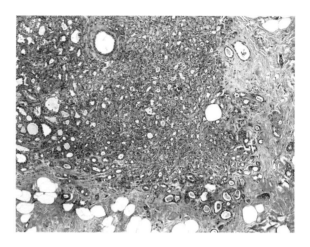

lesions. Sclerosing adenosis in associated with slightly increased risk for the subsequent development of invasive breast cancer, see Table 3.2.

Deciphering the Pathology Report

Again, the pathology report should be straightforward. If the reason for the biopsy was microcalcifications, their presence or absence should be mentioned. If the lesion is florid, the pathologist should identify it as such, because of the associated slightly increased risk for the development of cancer. Patients with a strong family history of breast cancer should be aware that the relative risk associated with this lesion is even higher, as it is with the other proliferative lesions with or without atypia.

Complex Sclerosing Lesion (Radial Scar)

Complex sclerosis lesions are stellate or "crab"-like in appearance and mimic the appearance of invasive cancer mammographically, by examination of the excised lesion with the unaided eye, and microscopically [8–10]. When the lesion is less than 1.0 cm, it is referred as a radial scar [9]. These lesions are characterized by a heterogeneous (mixed) proliferation of cells and stroma [9]. There is a central scar, which is comprised of a mixture of fibrous and elastic-like tissues, see Fig. 3.3. Acini are frequently present in the scar. Radiating fibrous connective tissue, ducts, and distorted lobules surround the central scar. Various degrees of hyperplasia can usually be seen at the periphery of the lesion. These lesions are not actually "scars" secondary to surgery or trauma. They are frequently found incidentally, but they can be visualized by mammography as well [8, 9, 11]. Complex sclerosing lesions convey a slightly increased risk for subsequent development with one caveat [4, 5]. If atypical ductal hyperplasia is present in these lesions, the risk is that of proliferative breast disease with atypia, see Table 3.2.

Fig. 3.3 Depicts a radial
scar with its "stellate"
outline, central fibroelastotic
core and radiating epithelial
cell components.

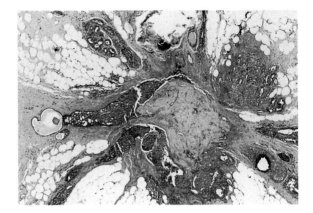

Deciphering the Pathology Report

An important thing to note in a pathology report of a complex sclerosing lesion (radial scar) is that if there is mention of atypical hyperplasia of any kind, the risk becomes that of the higher grade lesion.

Papilloma

Solitary papillomas are benign arborizing (tree like branching) neoplasms or tumors (clonal) with each "branch" containing a fibrous and vascular core or center covered by at least two cell layers, myoepithelial and luminal [9–11], see Fig. 3.4. Clonal refers to abnormal growths, comprised of cells that are genetically identical and is a feature of tumors or neoplasms, benign or malignant. Other descriptions for the gross (appearance to the unaided eye) lesion include "wart-like" and "cauliflower like." Solitary papillomas arise in large or lactiferous ducts and are usually attached to the duct wall by a stalk. They may twist or otherwise produce bloody nipple discharge.

Solitary papillomas are associated with a slightly increased risk of breast cancer [1–5, 9–11], see Table 3.2. Hyperplasia, atypical hyperplasia and ductal carcinoma can arise or be located in papillomas. The presence of hyperplasia alone would not be enough to change the risk category, but atypia and ductal carcinoma would increase the risk to the respective level risk associated with these lesions. A finding of atypia in a papillary lesion on a core needle warrants excision of the entire lesion to allow the pathologist to evaluate the entire lesion for more severe atypia or even presence of cancer, of spread of the proliferation beyond the duct's basement membrane, and evaluation of the surgical margins [9].

Multiple papillomas, sometimes referred to as papillomatosis, arise in the terminal ductal lobular units and are usually located peripherally in the breast [8–11]. They have the same general appearance as solitary papillomas but are smaller and multiple, see Fig. 3.5. It is generally reported that multiple papillomas are associated

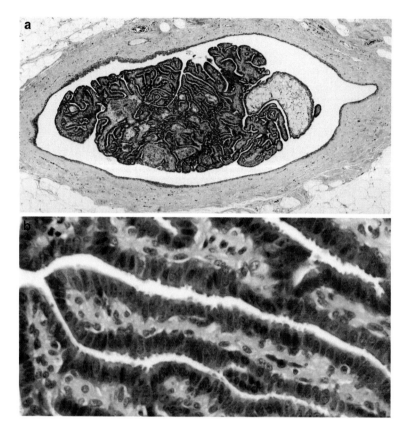

Fig. 3.4 (**a**) Shows a solitary intraductal papilloma with its arborizing, branch like projects covered with two cell layer – luminal and myoepithelial cells. (**b**) Illustrates the fibrovascular centers.

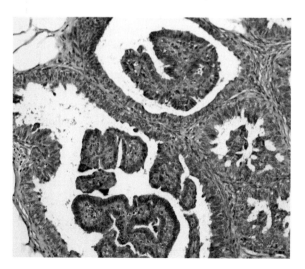

Fig. 3.5 Smaller papillomas or papillomatosis located in terminal ductal lobular units.

with the same degree of risk as a solitary papilloma; however, there is other data to suggest that the true risk for developing cancer for patients with multiple papillomas is somewhere in between that of proliferative breast disease without atypia and proliferative breast disease with atypia, i.e. atypical ductal hyperplasia [11]. These lesions are incidental findings.

Deciphering the Pathology Report

In solitary papilloma diagnosed by needle-core biopsy, careful attention to ascertain whether any atypia is present is important. If atypia is present, in most cases excision is warranted. In the case of excisional specimens, the pathology report should comment on the margins and whether or not there is any atypia. A diagnosis of papillomas without atypia warrants no further treatment, just awareness of the associated increased risk for cancer.

Atypical Ductal Hyperplasia

Atypical ductal hyperplasia differs from usual ductal hyperplasia in that there is architectural (arrangement of cells) and cytologic (cellular) atypia in addition to the hyperplasia [7, 8]. Atypical ductal hyperplasia is not usually clinically evident, and is usually an incidental finding, such as on a biopsy for mammographically detected microcalcifications. The median age of presentation is 50 years, with a range of 15–78 years. Atypical ductal hyperplasia tends to present at a slightly older age than usual ductal hyperplasia, and a slightly younger age than ductal carcinoma in situ. The incidence is increasing as a result of widespread screening mammography and advances in technology [9].

The cytologic features include monotonous cells with round nuclei and distinct cell (cytoplasmic) borders, compared to usual ductal hyperplasia without atypia. Small regular nucleoli can be present. Nucleoli are round, dense structures found in the nucleus and contain protein and RNA. Prominent and/or atypical nucleoli are associated usually with cancerous proliferations. Architecturally, the cells are more evenly spaced than in usual ductal hyperplasia without atypia. Some of the architectural patterns of growth include micropapillary (small papillary projections), solid, cribriform (the intraductal proliferation appears perforate like a sieve) patterns. In the cribriform or sieve-like pattern of atypical ductal hyperplasia, epithelium proliferates across the lumen to form "bridge-like structures", similar to those seen in ductal carcinoma in situ (DCIS), discussed in Chapter 4. In atypical hyperplasia, however, these bridge-like structures are not "rigid". The "rigid" bridge-like structures present in the DCIS are referred to as "Roman bridges" due to their resemblance to the sturdy arched bridges typical in Roman architecture, Fig. 3.6. The architectural and cytologic changes that characterize atypical ductal hyperplasia approach, but fall short of those required for ductal carcinoma in situ [7, 8], see Fig. 3.7.

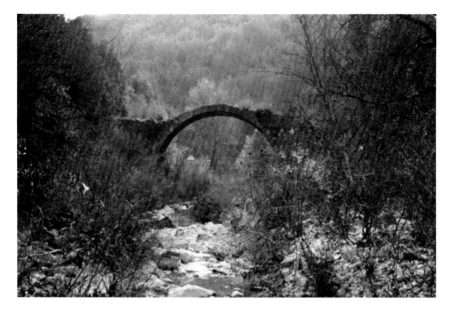

Fig. 3.6 Depicts the Ponte Della Pia bridge of Roman origin near the town of Rosia and the Castello di Spannochia – a "roman bridge." Legend has it that Pia de' Tolomei's ghost walks the bridge on nights when the moon is full dressed in white without touching her feet to the ground.

It can be difficult for the pathologist to decide where to draw the line between florid usual ductal hyperplasia without atypia, ductal hyperplasia with atypia and low grade ductal carcinoma in situ, especially on a core needle biopsy [7, 9]. To complicate matters these conditions can co-exist within the same biopsy and even the same terminal ductal lobular unit [9]. The architectural and cytological and cytologic features that define atypical ductal hyperplasia and in most cases separate it from florid usual ductal hyperplasia have some overlap with low grade DCIS. In some instances the distinction is difficult; but, neither is the biology likely to be that distinct for the two. In distinguishing atypical ductal hyperplasia and low grade DCIS, there is some agreement among breast pathology experts that size is important. Some feel that even if a lesion has all the features required for a diagnosis of low grade DCIS, a diagnosis of atypical ductal hyperplasia should be rendered if is not 2 mm in aggregate size or does not involve at least two entire to warrant a diagnosis of ductal carcinoma in situ [7–9]. Since size or extent of the atypical ductal proliferation cannot be determined on limited material, pathologists may use the following terminology: "atypical intraductal epithelial proliferation, or at least atypical ductal hyperplasia." A diagnosis of atypical ductal hyperplasia on a core needle biopsy that is not vacuum assisted should be followed by excision, because a reported 13–66% (average 36.5%) of core needle biopsy diagnoses will upgrade to a more significant lesion including invasive cancer on follow-up excisions [9].

A biopsy showing atypical hyperplasia alone carries an estimated relative risk of developing invasive cancer of about 4.0–5.0 that of the general population,

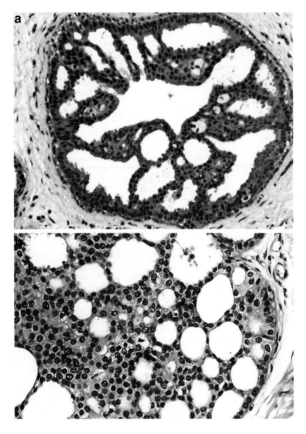

Fig. 3.7 (**a**) Atypical hyperplasia characterized by an intraductal proliferation of more uniform and more evenly distributed cells. The pattern is cribriform with tapered bridges across the lumen, round "punched out spaces" and occasionally irregular spaces and well. (**b**) Atypical hyperplasia with even more monotonous cells and regular, round holes, approaching ductal carcinoma in situ.

see Table 3.2. After a biopsy diagnosis of atypical ductal hyperplasia 3.7–22% of patients develop invasive carcinoma [8].

The genetic alterations reported for usual ductal hyperplasia suggest that it is a precursor of atypical ductal hyperplasia. Atypical ductal hyperplasia, in turn, has been shown to have many of the same mutations that are seen in ductal carcinoma and invasive cancer suggesting that atypical ductal hyperplasia is a precursor of these lesions [7, 8]. This evidence would support the theory that these proliferative lesions are on a continuum (from hyperplasia, to atypical hyperplasia, to carcinoma in situ) in the transformation (genetic alterations) and progression towards the uncontrolled cellular growth that defines cancer [7, 13, 14]

Excision is the usual therapy undertaken and may be all that is necessary; however, the risk of recurrent atypical ductal hyperplasia increases when present at the margin of excision. These patients may benefit from chemoprevention, especially if they have a strong family history, personal history, and/or inherited gene mutation.

Deciphering the Pathology Report

The diagnosis of atypical ductal hyperplasia requires further action, either surgery and/or chemoprevention. Sometimes, especially on core needle biopsy, the pathologist may see a lesion that is borderline between atypical hyperplasia and low grade ductal carcinoma in situ. There is not always a "bright line" separating the two entities. In these cases, the diagnosis may be more descriptive, such "atypical intraductal epithelial proliferation, cannot rule out a more serious lesion" with a comment that would suggest that an excision is necessary. Or, some pathologists may call such lesions borderline lesions or "borderline atypical intraductal epithelial proliferation." In any case, clinical and radiologic correlation and conservative excision are warranted. If the indication for biopsy was microcalcifications, again, the pathology report should mention their presence or absence. On excisional specimens, a statement about the margins should be in the report, i.e., whether the lesion was completely excised or whether the atypical ductal hyperplasia is at or close to a surgical margin. Measurement of the distance to the closest margin should be included.

Lobular Hyperplasia with Atypia

Atypical lobular hyperplasia is characterized by a proliferation of monotonous discohesive cells that partially fill or distend less than 50% of the acini within the lobule. The process can and often does extend along the ducts in what is termed a "pagetoid" fashion [15, 16]. Atypical lobular hyperplasia is associated with an increased risk for the development of invasive cancer (see Table 3.2). A diagnosis of atypical lobular hyperplasia requires no further action, unless it is extensive on a core needle biopsy [9]. Atypical lobular hyperplasia may also be referred to as lobular neoplasia, which is described further in Chap. 4.

Deciphering the Pathology Report

While reviewing the pathology report for atypical lobular hyperplasia, one must be aware that there is variable terminology. It can be referred to as lobular neoplasia. In that instance, communication with the pathologist must take place about the extent of the proliferation.

Flat Epithelial Atypia

Flat epithelial atypia is a lesion of the terminal ductal lobular unit. The terminal ductal lobular unit becomes enlarged and dilated and contain secretions and commonly microcalcifications [7, 8, 16, 17]. The spaces are lined by mildly atypical columnar

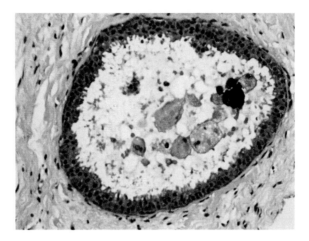

Fig. 3.8 Flat epithelial atypical characterized by a dilated round ductule that is lined by approximately three layers of mildly atypical cells with apical snouts. Ductal secretions and microcalcifications are present in the lumen.

(shaped like columns) epithelial cells that are in a single or 3–5 layers. The cells have pinched apical snouts (projections of cytoplasm on the top of the cells], see Fig. 3.8. These lesions are found incidentally and with increasing frequency with widespread use of screening mammography. The clinical significance of these lesions is not clearly defined, possibly in part due to the plethora of names that have been used to describe these lesions and the need for long-term follow-up data, see Table 3.2.

There is observational evidence that suggests that flat epithelial atypia may be neoplastic or preneoplastic [7, 8, 16, 17]. Flat epithelial atypias have often been seen in association with ductal carcinoma in situ and with some types of invasive cancers, specifically tubular carcinomas [16]. It has also been observed that the cells that make up similarly described lesions resemble the ductal carcinomas with which they are associated [16]. Flat epithelial atypias have been found to have molecular and genetic similarities with low-grade ductal carcinoma in situ and tubular carcinoma [16]. The clinical significance or associated risk for developing cancer after a diagnosis is not yet determined. Hence, the subsequent management of patients diagnosed with flat epithelial atypia, i.e., excision versus follow-up remains undertermined [18].

Deciphering the Pathology Report

As standardized criteria and terminology are being refined, tested and gradually adopted for what is most likely a spectrum of lesions, it would be important to realize that the entity described above could be designated by a variety of names other than flat epithelial atypia. A few examples include atypical cystic lobules, atypical cystic ducts, columnar cell change with atypia, columnar cell hyperplasia and ductal intraepithelial neoplasia of the flat monomorphic type, to name a few. Awareness of this fact is important. When a pathologist sees a lesion that she or he believes to be flat epithelial atypia, cutting deeper into the block for deeper sections to rule out a more serious associated lesion is recommended. The report may or may not indicate when deeper sections are examined. Most importantly the "triple test" should be applied, i.e., clinical, pathological, and radiologic correlation. If there are discrepancies between any of the three, further investigation is warranted. This is true for any pathologic diagnosis.

References

1. Non-cancerous breast conditions. http://www.cancer.org/docroot/CRI/content/CRI_2_6X_Non_Cancerous_Breast_Conditions_59.asp Accessed 7 Dec 2009
2. Dupont WE, Parl FF, Hartmann WH, Brinton LA, Winfield AC, Worrell JA, Schuler PA, Plummer WD (1993) Breast cancer risk associated with proliferative breast disease and atypical hyperplasia. Cancer 71(4):1258–1265
3. Collins LC, Baer HJ, Tamimi RM, Connonlly JL, Colditz GA, Schnitt SJ (2006) The influence of family history on breast cancer risk in women with biopsy-confirmed benign breast disease: results from the Nurses' Health Study. Cancer 107(6):1240–1247
4. Hartmann LC, Sellers TA, Frost MH, Lingle WL, Degnim AC, Ghosh K, Vierkant RA, Maloney SD et al (2005) Benign breast disease and the risk of breast cancer. N Engl J Med 353:229–237
5. London SJ, Connolly JL, Schnitt SH, Colditz GA (1992) A prospective study of benign breast disease and the risk of breast cancer. JAMA 267(7):941–944
6. Schnitt SJ (2003) The diagnosis and management of pre-invasive breast disease: flat epithelial atypia – classification, pathologic features and clinical significance. Breast Cancer Res 5:263–268
7. Rosen PP (2009) Ductal hyperplasia – usual and atypical. In: Rosen's breast pathology, 3rd edn. Pine, JW Jr., executive editor Lippincott Williams and Wilkins, Philadelphia, PA, pp 230–263
8. Tavassolli FA, Hoefler H, Rosai J, Holland R, Ellis IO, Schnitt SJ, Boecker W, Heywandg-Köbrunner SH (2003) Intraductal proliferative lesions. In: Tavassoli FA, Devilee P (eds) World Health Organization of tumors, pathology and genetics: tumors of the breast and female genital organs. IARC Press, Lyon, pp 63–73
9. Provenzano E, Pinder SE (2009) Pre-operative diagnosis of breast cancer in screening: problems and pitfalls. Pathology 41(1):3–17
10. Jacobs TW, Byrne C, Colditz G, Connolly JL, Schnitt S (1999) Radial scars in benign breast-biopsy specimens and the risk of breast cancer. N Engl J Med 340:430–436
11. Bussolati G, TavassoliFA, Nielsen BB, Ellis IO, MacGrogan G (2003) Benign epithelial proliferations. In: Tavassoli FA, Devilee P (eds) World Health Organization of tumors, pathology and genetics: tumors of the breast and female genital organs. IARC Press, Lyon, pp 81
12. Rosen PP (2009) Papilloma and related tumors. In Rosen's breast pathology, 3rd edn. Lippincott Williams and Wilkins, Philadelphia, PA, pp 85–104.
13. Gong G, DeVries S, Chew KL, Cha I, Ljung B-M, Waldman FM (2001) Genetic changes in paired atypical and usual ductal hyperplasia of the breast by comparative genomic hybridization. Clin Cancer Res (7) 2410–2414
14. Boecker W, Buerger H (2004) Usual and atypical ductal hyperplasia members of the same family? Curr Diagn Pathol 10:175–182
15. Ho BC, Tan PH (2009) Lobular neoplasia of the breast: 68 years on. Pathology 41(1):28–35
16. Contreras A, Sattar H (2009) Lobular neoplasia of the breast: an update. Arch Pathol Lab Med 133:1116–1120
17. Jara-Lazaro AR, Tse GM-N, Tan PH (2009) Columnar cells lesions of the breast: an update and significance on core biopsy. Pathology 41(1):18–27
18. Lerwill MF (2008) Flat epithelial atypia of the breast. Arch Pathol Lab Med 132:615–621
19. Piubello Q, Parisi A, Eccher A, Barbazeni G, Franchini Z, Iannucci A (2009) Flat epithelial atypia on cone needle biopsy: which is the right management? Am J Surg Pathol 33(7):1078–1084

Chapter 4
Precursor Lesions and Noninvasive Cancers

Joan Cangiarella and Fang Fan

Keywords Precursor lesions • Carcinoma in situ • Ductal carcinoma in situ (f) • Lobular neoplasia (f) • Atypical lobular hyperplasia • Lobular carcinoma in situ (f) • Relative risk • E-cadherin (f) • Non-obligate precursor • Loss of heterozygosity • Tumor suppressor gene • Type A lobular neoplasia • Type B lobular neoplasia • Ploidy • Estrogen receptor • Progesterone receptor • Magnetic resonance imaging (MRI) • Prophylactic mastectomy • Van Nuys grading system • Tamoxifen • Basement membrane • Micropapillary pattern • Cribriform pattern • Papillary pattern • Solid pattern • Comedo pattern

Lobular Neoplasia

Lobular neoplasia includes atypical lobular hyperplasia (ALH) and lobular carcinoma in situ (LCIS), and is characterized by a proliferation of uniform neoplastic epithelial cells within the terminal duct lobular unit with no extension beyond the basement membrane into the surrounding tissue, Table 4.1 [1]. The distinction between ALH and LCIS is based on the extent of epithelial proliferation. In LCIS the epithelial proliferation fills the acini of the terminal duct lobular unit, Figs. 4.1 and 4.2. Proliferations that partially fill the acini are designated as ALH. The appearance of the cells that comprise these lesions is identical.

There are arguments for and against lumping ALH and LCIS together as lobular neoplasia, such as the differences in relative risk for development of cancer between the two entities, 5.5 times the relative risk for ALH and 8–10 times the relative risk for LCIS. Arguments in favor of categorizing ALH and LCIS together as lobular neoplasia were supported by observations that cancer risk was relatively equal for either breast, the time interval between a diagnosis of lobular neoplasia and the subsequent invasive cancer was long, and the fact that the invasive cancer could be either ductal or lobular in type.

J. Cangiarella (✉)
Associate Professor, Department of Pathology, New York University School of Medicine, New York, NY, USA
e-mail: joan.cangiarella@nymc.org

P.A. Thomas (ed.), *Breast Cancer and its Precursor Lesions*, Current Clinical Pathology, DOI 10.1007/978-1-60327-154-7_4, © Springer Science+Business Media, LLC 2011

Table 4.1 Terminology

Lobular carcinoma in situ (LCIS) is the result of proliferation of uniform,
  discohesive epithelial cells within terminal ducts or acini of lobules

Lobules have more than 50% of ductules completely filled

Enlargement of lobules not necessary, and only one lobule may be affected

Atypical lobular hyperplasia (ALH) is the proliferation of similar cells as LCIS,
  but acini are partially filled

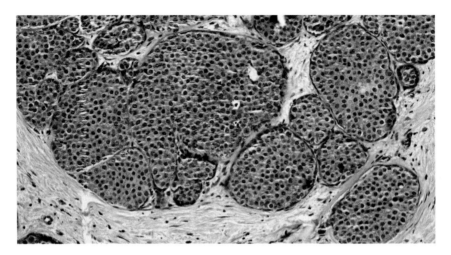

Fig. 4.1 The lobules are distended by a proliferation of small uniform cells.

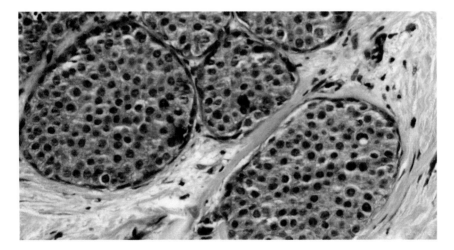

Fig. 4.2 The cells are monotonous with small, round uniform nuclei.

Based on the same observations that supported the concept of lobular neoplasia, this spectrum of lesions was only considered an indicator of increased risk for the subsequent development of cancer. However, recent advances in molecular and genetic techniques and studies of long-term follow-up call to question this concept and suggest that lobular neoplasia may instead be an indolent or non-obligate (not fully committed) precursor to invasive cancer [2–4]. For example, while carcinoma can develop in either breast after a diagnosis of lobular neoplasia, in the majority of patients subsequent carcinomas developed in the same site as the initial lesion [5] and the invasive cancer was much more likely to be of lobular type. Other evidence comes from analysis of the E-cadherin gene. E-cadherin is a cell surface adhesion molecule normally present on all epithelial cells Fig. 4.3. Adhesion molecules bind

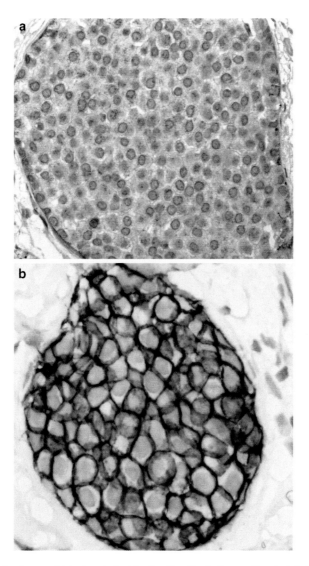

Fig. 4.3 (**a**) An immunohistochemical stain for E-cadherin is negative in lobular neoplasia. (**b**) An immunohistochemical stain for E-cadherin in an intraductal proliferation.

cells to each other and the basement membrane. The loss or down-regulation of E-cadherin is a molecular feature of both lobular neoplasia and invasive lobular carcinomas [6] and is likely responsible for the discohesive nature of the cells that comprise lobular neoplasia. Mutations in the E-cadherin gene that are identified in invasive lobular carcinomas have also been demonstrated in adjacent foci of LCIS [7]. Molecular studies show a lack of E-cadherin reactivity in both LCIS and invasive lobular carcinomas [8]. Recent studies have suggested genomic clonality (genetically identical cells, a property of cancers) in paired samples from patients with synchronous LCIS and invasive lobular carcinoma with the most frequent alterations being gain of 1q and loss of 16q [9]. Chromosomes, which are all assigned numbers, have two rod shaped or strand like DNA "arms", one long and one short. The long arm is designated by the letter "q" beside the chromosome number. The short arm of a chromosome is designated by the letter "p". The loss of heterozygosity on chromosome 16 q the locus for E-cadherin gene, was detected in 30% of LCIS cases in one study [4]. Heterozygosity refers to the fact that two genes occupy the same position or locus on each side or arm of a chromosome are different. Loss of the different gene in this case suggests that the gene loss was a tumor suppressor gene, i.e. a gene that in non-cancerous tissues suppresses the development of cancer. Simultaneous loss of E-cadherin and catenins have been described in lobular carcinoma in situ and in invasive lobular carcinomas suggesting that the loss of E-cadherin expression may be an important step associated with the formation of lobular carcinoma in situ as a precursor of invasive lobular cancer [10]. LCIS has also been shown to be associated with areas of microinvasion [11]. Additionally, recent studies have shown LCIS and synchronous (occurring at the same time) invasive lobular carcinoma possess similar genetic profiles, supporting the notion that lobular neoplasia is a direct precursor to invasive lobular carcinoma [12]. Over the next decade with the advancement of molecular information we can hope for a deeper understanding of the mechanisms of lobular neoplasia leading to better long term management and treatment of these lesions.

Clinical Presentation

Lobular neoplasia is most often discovered as an incidental microscopic finding in a breast specimen removed for another reason. There are no clinical findings, no palpable mass, and in most cases no signs by mammography, Table 4.2. The true incidence and prevalence are difficult to predict due to the lack of clinical and

Table 4.2 Clinical Presentation	Incidental finding
	No clinical or mammographic findings
	Low incidence but increasing
	Mainly in premenopausal women
	High rate of multicentricity and bilaterality

mammographic findings associated with lobular neoplasia, but the incidence is increasing [13]. Lobular neoplasia can be found in both pre- and post-menopausal patients. Characteristically, LCIS is multifocal, multicentric (different quadrants of the breast) and bilateral. Multicentricity has been seen in 42–86% of cases and bilaterality in 9–69% [14].

Risk Factors and Diagnosis

The most notable risk factor for the development of lobular neoplasia is a family history of mammary cancer [15].

At biopsy the main problem is the distinction between lobular neoplasia and low-grade ductal carcinoma in situ (DCIS). Immunohistochemical staining for E- cadherin is useful in this regard with negativity in most cases of LCIS and positivity in cases of DCIS.

Lobular neoplasia may be classified according to nuclear size into small cell or large cell types. The classic type is designated as type A cells and are small and uniform with scant cytoplasm and round central nuclei, which lack nucleoli, Table 4.3. The larger cell type or type B cells (pleomorphic) have larger and less uniform nuclei, occasional nucleoli, and more abundant cytoplasm.

Lobular carcinoma in situ (LCIS) deserves further discussion as a distinct entity. Pleomorphic LCIS is a recently described variant with cells similar to type B LCIS but are characterized by more pleomorphism, larger nuclei, and distinct nucleoli [16]. Central necrosis with calcification can occur. This variant differs from classic LCIS in that the majority present with a mammographic abnormality, i.e. a mass or calcification. Pleomorphic LCIS may show a biological behavior similar to DCIS with the current recommended treatment for pleomorphic lobular carcinoma in situ similar to DCIS i.e. excision with free margins with or without radiation therapy [16].

The presence of intracytoplasmic mucin vacuoles has been described in LCIS and may result in signet ring cells, so called because these cells resemble a finger ring bearing an engraved signet. The signet ring appearance is due to compression of the nucleus to one side by cytoplasmic mucin. The presence of these mucinous vacuoles is uncommon in ductal carcinoma and favors a diagnosis of LCIS. A pagetoid pattern of growth of neoplastic cells of LCIS or ALH from the lobular ductule along the ductal epithelium may also be reported.

Table 4.3 Diagnosis

Classic type, small cells (Type A)
Rare large type, more pleomorphic (Type B)
Pleomorphic lobular type, associated with necrosis and calcification, treated like DCIS
Signet ring cells seen
Molecular studies: ER/PR +, C-erb-2 negative, p53 negative, E-cadherin negative

On fine needle aspiration biopsy the diagnosis of LCIS is difficult to distinguish from ALH or ductal carcinoma in situ [17]. The presence of intracytoplasmic lumina within cells and the presence of small cell groups similar to the acini of LCIS are helpful cytologic features [17]. Cells arranged in single file should also suggest a lobular lesion; in this instance suspicious for invasive lobular. Aspiration smears from cases of LCIS may be indistinguishable from invasive lobular carcinoma [18].

Most cells of LCIS are positive for estrogen and progesterone receptor and negative for C-erb-2 [19, 20] and p53 [21]. Ploidy (the number of homologous chromosome sets) in cell studies of LCIS show the majority to be DNA diploid (two sets of chromosomes) [19, 20].

Implications and Relationship to Malignancy

As mentioned above, lobular neoplasia is associated with an increased risk of breast cancer bilaterally. The development of carcinoma is often 10–20 years after the initial diagnosis of LCIS [22–25]. Studies with follow-up periods of 14–24 years have shown that approximately 12–30% of patients with a diagnosis of LCIS will eventually develop an invasive cancer, Table 4.4 [1, 22–24, 26]. Most studies have shown that the relative risk of developing an invasive cancer after a diagnosis of LCIS is increased approximately 7–12 times above the general population [1, 22, 23]. Invasive carcinomas are equally as likely to occur in the opposite or contralateral breast as in the ipsilateral breast [27] and majority of cancers are of the invasive ductal type. In more recent studies with periods of follow-up from 4 to 7 years, recurrence rates range from 6 to 9% with over 60% being invasive carcinomas, many of the ductal type [20, 28, 29].

Implications for Management

Most current treatments are based on the belief that lobular neoplasia is a risk factor for the development of invasive carcinoma rather than a true precursor. As the majority of women with lobular neoplasia will not develop cancer and of those who do the risk is approximately equal for both breasts, the consensus is to treat lobular neoplasia with careful observation. Observation must be life-long as the risk remains indefinitely.

Table 4.4 Implications and relationship to malignancy for LCIS

Increased risk of breast cancer for long follow-up periods
Relative risk of 7–12× over general population
Risk is approximately equal for both breasts

Patients who chose observation require yearly physical examinations and usually a yearly mammogram. The role of magnetic resonance imaging (MRI) in high-risk patients is currently under investigation. Radiation therapy appears to have no role at this time.

There are few guidelines and no consensus for the recommended treatment of patients with lobular neoplasia diagnosed on percutaneous core biopsy. The diagnosis of LCIS at core needle biopsy is uncommon, representing 0.3% of needle core biopsies in a multi-institutional series of over 32,000 biopsies [30]. In most series, the finding of LCIS on core biopsy leads to surgical excision [31, 32]. Some recommend excisional biopsy when the diagnosis of LCIS is associated with a mass [33]. Others find excision unnecessary but this is the minority [34]. Radiologic/pathologic agreement is important. If there is discordance between the two, excision is recommended. A summary of several studies showed a core biopsy diagnosis of LCIS led to a cancer at excision in approximately 22% of cases [35]. On this basis, excision would be recommended for most patients. One recent study noted the extent or amount of LCIS on core biopsy was important with diffuse LCIS (defined as greater than one lobule per core) being associated with a greater risk of invasive carcinoma [36]. Ongoing studies may lead to guidelines for management of LCIS at percutaneous biopsy, but it has been reported that for patients who have lobular neoplasia on needle core biopsy end up having a more significant lesion on excision and the likelihood of this upstaging increases with the extent of the lobular neoplasia.

A bilateral prophylactic mastectomy is considered only in patients who do not want to bear the risk associated with LCIS or in those patients with other significant risks for breast cancer, i.e. strong family history or history of BRCA mutations. Most physicians consider this therapy drastic for the management of LCIS.

For patients with LCIS, Tamoxifen reduces the risk of invasive cancer by 56% thus chemoprevention is an option for some patients [37]. Raloxifene has also been shown to reduce the risk of developing invasive breast cancer in postmenopausal women with LCIS [38].

For patients with invasive breast cancer who have been treated with conservative surgery and radiation the presence and extent of LCIS in the tissue surrounding a lumpectomy has not been shown to affect the risk of local recurrence in patients in most studies, Table 4.5 [39, 40].

Table 4.5 Implications for management

A diagnosis of lobular neoplasia requires lifelong surveillance
For most patients, a diagnosis of LCIS on percutaneous biopsy will require surgical excision
A bilateral prophylactic mastectomy now is felt to be an extreme intervention reserved for special circumstances
Tamoxifen or Raloxifene have reduced the risk of invasive cancer and are options for some

Deciphering the Pathology Report

Since LCIS is mainly an incidental finding no specific gross alterations are described in the pathology report. The extent of the LCIS or ALH found on a core biopsy should be mentioned in the pathology report. The presence of LCIS at an operative or excision margin is not relevant and does not warrant re-excision.

The finding of LCIS in a percutaneous core biopsy or a fine-needle aspiration biopsy warrants excision in most cases. The finding of LCIS in a surgical biopsy warrants lifelong surveillance.

Ductal Carcinoma In Situ

Ductal carcinoma in situ (DCIS) is an intraductal lesion characterized by proliferation of cancerous cells confined within ducts and lobules with no evidence of invasion through basement membrane into surrounding stroma (Fig. 4.4). That being said, DCIS is considered a precursor lesion for invasive breast carcinoma. DCIS can be a non-obligate precursor (not committed to progression) or an obligate precursor (if left untreated is committed to progress to invasive cancer) depending on the grade. DCIS is associated with increased risk (relative risk 8.0–11.0×) of developing invasive carcinoma in the same breast compared to the general population [41, 42].

The incidence of DCIS has increased since 1983, mainly due to the introduction of screening mammograms and the increased public awareness of breast cancer [43]. DCIS now accounts for 20% of mammographically detected breast cancers [44].

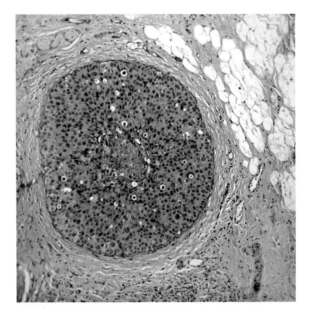

Fig. 4.4 Ductal carcinoma in-situ. Ducts are distended and filled with monotonous proliferation of tumor cells. But the basement membrane around the ducts is intact.

Clinical Presentation

The majority of DCIS present as mammographic abnormalities. They are most frequently associated with microcalcifications, soft tissue abnormalities or architectural distortion. A small percentage of patients may have a palpable abnormality or nipple discharge. Up to 5% are detected incidentally in surgical specimens for unrelated reasons.

Risk Factors and Diagnosis

The risk factors for DCIS are similar to that for invasive carcinoma and include family history, presence of proliferative breast disease, genetic factors, among others. See Chap. 5 for more details.

The diagnosis is usually made on core needle biopsy or excisional biopsy. Fine needle aspiration of breast alone cannot reliably differentiate DCIS from invasive carcinoma.

Deciphering the Pathology Report

The final pathology report for DCIS should include factors currently considered to be important in predicting risk for local recurrence or progression to invasive carcinoma or selection of treatment protocol. Many studies have shown that there is a relationship between histologic features of DCIS and clinical outcome, including time to development of invasive cancer and local recurrence after excision. However, there is still no universal agreement on the classification/grading of DCIS[45, 46]. The Lagios, Van Nuys and European systems all recognize three main categories that are equivalent to low, intermediate, and high-grade, low-grade comprising those lesions that most resemble their non-tumor counterparts in the breast and having the best potential outcomes and high-grade representing those in-situ carcinomas that least resemble their benign cells of origin and are associated with the worst potential outcomes. Intermediate-grade, as would be expected in between the two in appearance and behavior. The latest World Health Organization (WHO) book on Tumors of the Breast and Female Genital Organs also recommend a three-tiered grading system to divide DCIS into low, intermediate and high-grade based primarily on cellular/nuclear features and/or necrosis [47].

There are five major architectural patterns in DCIS including comedo, cribriform, micropapillary, papillary, and solid (Fig. 4.5). There should be a comment about which pattern is present in the pathology report. DCIS with comedo pattern

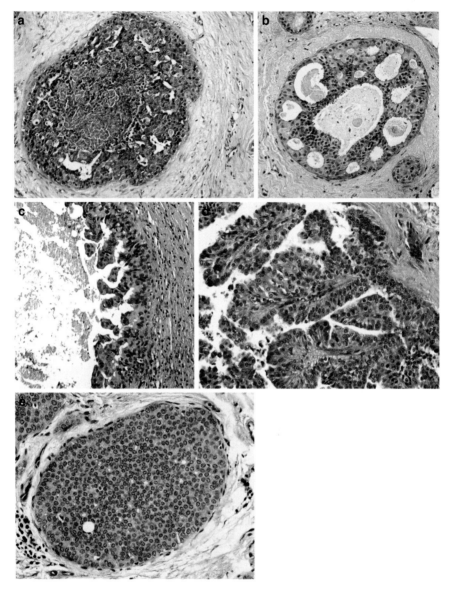

Fig. 4.5 Ductal carcinoma in-situ. (**a**) Comedo pattern. There is central comedo necrosis and surround tumor cells have high nuclear grade. (**b**) Cribriform pattern. (**c**) Micropapillary pattern. (**d**) Papillary pattern. (**e**) Solid pattern.

is associated with a high local recurrence rate after excision. The micropapillary pattern may be associated with more extensive multi-quadrant disease.

The important characteristics of DCIS are summarized in Table 4.6. The features of DCIS that should be included in the final pathology report are listed in Table 4.7

Table 4.6 Important characteristics of ductal carcinoma in-situ

Intraductal proliferation of neoplastic cells with no invasion into surrounding stroma

Present as

  − Mammographic abnormalities
  − Palpable abnormalities
  − Nipple discharge
  − Incidental

Precursor for invasive carcinoma

Five major architectural patterns

  − Comedo
  − Cribriform
  − Solid
  − Papillary
  − Micropapillary

Three histologic grades

  − Low-grade
  − Intermediate-grade
  − High-grade

Table 4.7 Important features of ductal carcinoma in-situ included in pathology report

Nuclear grade

Necrosis

Overall grade

Architectural pattern

Size/extent of the lesion

Margin status

Microcalcifications

Correlation with the histologic and mammographic findings if available

Expression of biomarkers including ER, PR and Her-2/neu

References

1. Haagensen CD, Lane N, Lattes R, Bodian C (1978) Lobular neoplasia (so-called lobular carcinoma in situ) of the breast. Cancer 42:737–739
2. Sapino A, Frigerio A, Peterse JL, Arisio R, Collucia C, Bussolati G (2000) Mammographically detected in situ lobular carcinoma of the breast. Virchows Arch 436:421–430
3. Nayar R, Zhuang Z, Merino MJ, Silverberg SG (1997) Loss of heterozygosity on chromosome 11q13 in lobular lesions of the breast using microdissection and polymerase chain reaction. Hum Pathol 28:277–282
4. Lakhani S, Zhuang Z, Sloane J, Stratton M (1995) Loss of heterozygosity in lobular carcinoma in situ of the breast. Mol Pathol 48:M74–M78
5. Fisher ER, Land SR, Fisher B, Mamounas E, Gilarski L, Wolmark N (2004) Pathologic findings from the National Surgical Adjuvant Breast and Bowel Project: twelve-year observations concerning lobular carcinoma in situ. Cancer 100:238–244
6. Hanby AM, Hughes TA (2008) In situ and invasive lobular neoplasia of the breast. Histopathology 52:58–66

7. Vos CB, Cleton-Jansen AM, Berx G et al (1997) E-cadherin inactivation in lobular carcinoma in situ of the breast: an early event in tumorigenesis. Br J Cancer 76:1131–1133

8. Acs G, Lawton TS, Rebbeck TR, LiVolsi VA, Shang PJ (2001) Differential expression of E-cadherin in lobular and ductal neoplasms of the breast and its biologic and diagnostic implications. Am J Clin Pathol 115:85–98

9. Hwang ES, Nyante SJ, Chen YY, Moore D, DeVries S, Korkola JE, Esserman LJ, Waldman FM (2004) Clonality of lobular carcinoma in situ and synchronous invasive lobular carcinoma. Cancer 100:2562–2572

10. De Leeuw WJF, Vos CBJ, Peterse JL, De Vijver MJ, Litvinov S, Van Roy F Cornelisse CJ, Cleton-Jansen AM. (1997) Simultaneous loss of E-cadherin and catenins in invasive lobular breast cancer and lobular carcinoma in situ. J Pathol 183:404–411

11. Nemoto T, Castillo N, Tsukada Y et al (1998) Lobular carcinoma in situ with microinvasion. J Surg Oncol 67:41–46

12. Lerwill MF (2006) The evolution of lobular neoplasia. Adv Anat Pathol 13:157–165

13. Li CI, Anderson BO, Daling JR, Moe RE (2002) Changing incidence of lobular carcinoma in situ of the breast. Breast Cancer Res Treat 75:259–268

14. Nielsen M (1989) Autopsy studies of the occurrence of cancerous, atypical and benign epithelial lesions in the female breast. APMIS 97:20–26

15. Claus EB, Stowe M, Carter D (2003) Family history of breast and ovarian cancer and the risk of breast carcinoma in situ. Breast Cancer Res Treat 78:7–15

16. Sneige N, Wang J, Baker B, Krishnamurthy S, Middleton L (2002) Clinical, histopathologic, and biologic features of pleomorphic lobular (ductal-lobular) carcinoma in situ of the breast: a report of 24 cases. Mod Pathol 15:1044–1050

17. Ustun M, Berner A, Davidson B, Risberg B (2002) Fine-needle aspiration cytology of lobular carcinoma in situ. Diagn Cytopathol 27:22–26

18. Silverman JF, Masood S, Ducatman BS, Wang HH, Sneige N (1993) Can FNA biopsy separate atypical hyperplasia, carcinoma in situ and invasive carcinoma of the breast? Cytomorphologic criteria and limitations in diagnosis. Diagn Cytopathol 9:713–728

19. Ottesen GL, Graversen HP, Blichert-Toft M, Christensen IJ, Andersen JA (2000) Carcinoma in situ of the female breast. 10 year follow-up results of a prospective nationwide study. Breast Cancer Res Treat 62:197–210

20. Fisher ER, Costantino J, Fisher B, Palekar AS (1996) Pathologic findings from the National Surgical Adjuvant Breast Project (NASBP) Protocol B-17: five year observations concerning lobular carcinoma in situ. Cancer 78:1403–1416

21. Albonico G, Querzoli P, Ferretti S, Rinaldi R, Nemci I (1998) Biological profile of in situ breast cancer investigated by immunohistochemical technique. Cancer Detect Prev 22:313–318

22. Rosen PP, Kosloff CC, Lieberman PH, Adair F, Braun DW Jr (1978) Lobular carcinoma in situ of the breast. Detailed analysis of 99 patients with average follow-up of 24 years. Am J Surg Pathol 2:225–251

23. Page DL, Kidd TJ, Dupont WD, Simpson JF, Rogers LW (1991) Lobular neoplasia of the breast: higher risk for subsequent invasive cancer predicted by more extensive disease. Hum Pathol 22:1232–1239

24. Wheeler JE, Enterline HT, Roseman JM, Tomasulo JP, McIlvaine CH, Fitts WT Jr, Kirshenbaum J (1974) Lobular carcinoma in situ of the breast. Long-term follow-up. Cancer 34:554–563

25. Frykberg ER, Bland KI (1994) Management of in situ and minimally invasive breast carcinoma. World J Surg 18:45–57

26. Page DL, Dupont WD, Rogers LW et al (1985) Atypical hyperplastic lesions of the female breast. A long-term follow-up study of cancer risk. Cancer 55:2698–2708

27. Millikan R, Dressler L, Geradts J, Graham M (1995) The need for epidemiologic studies of in situ carcinoma of the breast. Breast Cancer Res Treat 35:65–77

28. Zurida S, Bartoli C, Galimberti V, Raselli R, Barletta L (1996) Interpretation of the risk associated with the unexpected finding of lobular carcinoma in situ. Ann Surg Oncol 3:57–61

29. Carson W, Sanchez-Forgach E, Stomper P, Penetrante R, Tsangaris TN, Edge SB (1994) Lobular carcinoma in situ: observation without surgery as an appropriate therapy. Ann Surg Oncol 1:141–146

30. Lechner MC, Jackman RJ, Brem RF, Evans WP, Parker SH, Smid AP (1999) Lobular carcinoma in situ and atypical lobular hyperplasia at percutaneous biopsy with surgical correlation: a multi-institutional study (abstr). Radiology 213:106
31. Elsheikh TM, Silverman JF (2005) Follow-up surgical excision is indicated when breast core needle biopsies show atypical lobular hyperplasia or lobular carcinoma in situ: a correlative study of 33 patients with review of the literature. Am J Surg Pathol 29:534–543
32. Foster MC, Helvie MA, Gregory NE, Rebner M, Nees AV, Paramagul C (2004) Lobular carcinoma in situ or atypical lobular hyperplasia at core-needle biopsy: is excisional biopsy necessary? Radiology 231:813–819
33. Middleton LP, Shakeitha G, Stephens T, Stelling CB, Sneige N, Sahin AA (2003) Lobular carcinoma in situ diagnosed by core needle biopsy: when should it be excised? Mod Pathol 16:120–129
34. Renshaw AA, Cartegna N, Derhagopia RP, Gould EW (2002) Lobular neoplasia in breast core needle biopsy specimens is not associated with an increased risk of ductal carcinoma in situ or invasive carcinoma. Am J Clin Pathol 117:797–799
35. Cohen MA (2004) Cancer upgrades at excisional biopsy after diagnosis of atypical lobular hyperplasia or lobular carcinoma in situ at core-needle biopsy: some reasons why. Radiology 231:617–621
36. Esserman LE, Lamea L, Tanev S, Poppiti R (2007) Should the extent of lobular neoplasia on core biopsy influence the decision for excision? Breast J 13:55–61
37. Fisher B, Costantino JP, Wickerham L et al (1998) Tamoxifen for prevention of breast cancer report of the National Surgical Adjuvant Breast and Bowel Project P-1 Study. J Natl Cancer Inst 90:1371–1388
38. Vogel VG, Constantino JP, Wickerham DL, Cronin WM, Cecchini RS Atkins JN et al, National Surgical Adjuvant Breast and Bowel Project (NSABP) (2006) Effects of tamoxifen vs. raloxifene on the risk of developing invasive breast cancer and other disease outcomes: the NSABP Study of tamoxifen and raloxifene (STAR) P-2 trial. JAMA 295:2727–2741
39. Abner AL, Connolly JL, Recht A, Bornstein B, Nixon A, Hetelekidis S, Silver B, Harris JR, Schnitt SJ (2000) The relation between the presence and extent of lobular carcinoma in situ and the risk of local recurrence for patients with infiltrating carcinoma of the breast treated with conservative surgery and radiation therapy. Cancer 88:1072–1077
40. Stolier AJ, Barre G, Bolton JS, Fuhrman G, Looney S (2004) Breast conservation therapy for invasive lobular carcinoma: the impact of lobular carcinoma in situ in the surgical specimen on local recurrence and axillary node status. Am Surg 70:818–821
41. Dupont WD, Page DL (1985) Risk factors for breast cancer in women with proliferative breast disease. N Engl J Med 312:146–151
42. Fitzgibbons PL, Henson DE, Hutter RV (1998) Benign breast changes and the risk for subsequent breast cancer: an update of the 1985 consensus statement. Cancer Committee of the College of American Pathologists. Arch Pathol Lab Med 122:1053–1055
43. Ernster VL, Barclay J, Kerlikowske K, Wilkie H, Ballard-Barbash R (2000) Mortality among women with ductal carcinoma in situ of the breast in the population-based surveillance, epidemiology and end results program. Arch Intern Med 160:953–958
44. Evans AJ, Pinder SE, Ellio IO, Wilson AR (2001) Screen detected ductal carcinoma in situ (DCIS): overdiagnosis or an obligate precursor of invasive disease? J Med Screen 8:149–151
45. The Consensus Conference Committee (1997) Consensus Conference on the classification of ductal carcinoma in situ. Cancer 80:1798–1802
46. Leonard GD, Swain SM (2004) Ductal carcinoma in situ, complexities and challenges. J Natl Cancer Inst 96:906–920
47. Tavassoli FA, Hoefler H, Rosai J et al (2003) Intraductal proliferative lesions. In: Tavassoli FA, Devilee P (eds) Pathology and genetics: tumors of the breast and female genital organs. IARC Press, Lyon, pp 63–73

Chapter 5
Breast Cancer

Fang Fan

Keywords Cancer • Stage • Histologic type • Grade • Hormonal status • Invasive ductal carcinoma, not otherwise specified (f) • Invasive lobular carcinoma (f) • Estrogen receptor • Progesterone receptor • Her-2/neu • Terminal duct lobular unit • Desmoplastic • Scirrhous • Paget's disease • Inflammatory carcinoma • Medullary carcinoma • Peau de' orange • BRCA1 • BRCA2 • Li Fraumeni syndromel • Cowden syndrome • Racial influences • Obesity • Bloom and Richardson grading system • Tubulolobular pattern • Pleomorphic variant • Tubular carcinoma (f) • Mucinous carcinoma (f) • Medullary carcinoma (f) • Invasive papillary carcinoma • Apocrine carcinoma • Metaplastic carcinoma

Invasive Ductal Carcinoma

Invasive ductal carcinoma (cancer) refers to a malignant epithelial proliferation which stems from the terminal duct-lobular unit. These tumors are so-named because of the resemblance of the tumor cells to the cells normally lining the ducts as opposed to the lobules. These invasive epithelial tumor cells are no longer surrounded by a myoepithelial or basal cell layer as in the normal duct, and the basement membrane is lost as well. The series of complex interactions between the epithelial cells and the basement membrane and surrounding stroma which allows them to develop this capacity to invade are beyond the scope of this book, but suffice it to say that the interactions are among the most elusive and studied relationships in all of cancer biology.

Invasive ductal carcinoma classified as "no special type (NST)" or "not otherwise specified (NOS)" is the largest category of invasive breast cancer, see Fig. 5.1. Invasive ductal carcinoma, NST accounts for 47–80% of all invasive lesions, depending on the population studied. This type of carcinoma shows a growth pattern in which at

F. Fan (✉)
Associate Professor, Department of Pathology and Laboratory Medicine,
University of Kansas Medical Center, Kansas City, KS, USA
e-mail: ffan@kumc.edu

P.A. Thomas (ed.), *Breast Cancer and its Precursor Lesions*, Current Clinical Pathology, DOI 10.1007/978-1-60327-154-7_5, © Springer Science+Business Media, LLC 2011

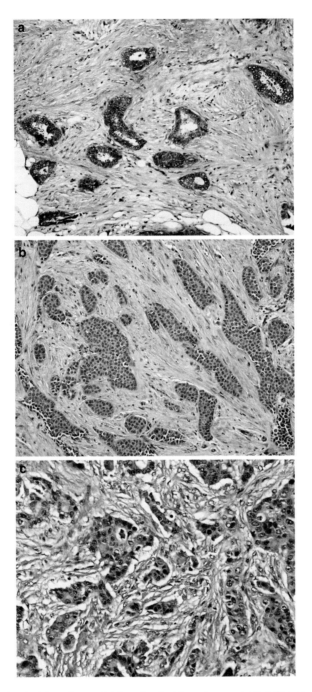

Fig. 5.1 Invasive ductal carcinoma. (**a**) Invasive ductal carcinoma, grade I. Tumor cells have low nuclear grade and the majority of them form tubules. (**b**) Invasive ductal carcinoma, grade II. Tumor cells form solid cords and trabeculae with intermediate nuclear grade. (**c**) Invasive ductal carcinoma, grade III. Tumor cells do not form tubules and have high nuclear grade with frequent mitoses.

least some cells show an attempt to form some resemblance to a ductal structure. This type often shows a desmoplastic (fibrotic) stromal reaction to the invasive epithelial cells, forming a hard or "scirrhous" tumor nodule, hence the older terminology "scirrhous carcinoma."

Clinical Presentation

Breast cancer often presents as a mass discovered by a woman during breast self-examination. During these times of more aggressive screening, it is also often discovered as a mammographic abnormality such as an irregular density or calcification. It can also present as an incidental finding on biopsy for another lesion, such as ductal carcinoma in situ (also often performed due to microcalcification). Cancers of the breast can cause irregularities in the skin, such as a peculiar thickening resembling the peel of an orange known as "peau d'orange," and skin fixation to underlying tissue with puckering. When the dermal lymphatics are involved by carcinoma as sometimes occurs with advanced disease, there is erythema and warmness of the skin overlying the breast. This condition is referred to as "inflammatory carcinoma." Nipple changes can also occur, such as inversion or retraction. Paget's disease presents as an eczema-like ulceration and crusting of the skin of the nipple and/or areola, due to the invading carcinoma cells. Less commonly, a palpable lymph node in the axilla or supraclavicular area can alert a clinician to a previously undiscovered primary breast malignancy.

The most common location of a carcinoma of the breast is the upper outer quadrant, where 50% of tumors present. The remaining quadrants are each involved in about 10%, and the subareolar area is the initial site of presentation in 20% of tumors. Cancers of the left breast are slightly more common than the right, for unknown reasons.

The incidence of carcinoma increases with advancing age, being rare before 25 years of age, increasing steadily until reaching an incidence of 1 in 29 in the seventh decade. The overall incidence has been fairly steady since 1988.

Risk Factors and Diagnosis

Family history is a well known risk factor for breast cancer, with an estimated 5–10% of cases attributable to inheritance of an autosomal (any chromosome other than a sex chromosome) dominant gene [1]. History of breast cancer in a first degree relative is especially significant, with an estimated relative risk of 2–3 times that of the general population. The risk is greatest for relatives of patients with premenopausal cancers and cancers involving both breasts (bilateral), increasing up to 9 times that of the general population. Certain genetic mutations have been implicated, among the more important of which are BRCA1 and BRCA2 gene mutations [2]. These two genes account for about 20% of familial cases, and have been found to increase the risk of ovarian cancers as well. Breast cancer is associated with less common mutations such as abnormalities in DNA repair that results in ataxia-telangiectasia. Breast cancer can also be associated with syndromes which carry increased risk of many different kinds of cancers such as Li-Fraumeni and Cowden syndromes.

Regarding racial influences, white women have a higher overall breast cancer incidence than black women; however black women tend to present with higher stage tumors and have poorer overall survival than whites. This is in part due to disparities in access to health care and screening, disparities in treatment, but there is increasing evidence that biology may also play a role [3]. For example, contrary to post-menopausal cancer incidence, black women under 40 years of age are more often diagnosed with breast cancer than whites under 40, and their cancers tend to have higher nuclear grade, and less often express hormone receptors than the cancers in whites. Also, certain mutations have been found to be different in blacks than whites [4].

Previous or current carcinoma in the opposite breast or endometrium carry an increased risk of breast cancer, as does proliferative breast disease such as usual ductal hyperplasia (1.5 times relative risk), atypical ductal hyperplasia (4–5 times relative risk), and ductal carcinoma in situ (8–10 times relative risk).

Hormones are known risk factors for breast cancer [5]. This makes sense when one considers the large percentage of breast cancers that carry receptors for estrogen and progesterone. Among these risks are never having borne a child (nulliparity), older age at first pregnancy, and early menarche/late menopause. Each of these factors suggests a longer exposure to menstrual cycles without the "break" provided by pregnancy or later menarche/earlier menopause. Effects of exogenous estrogens from oral contraceptives or postmenopausal hormone therapy are controversial – the jury is still out. The risk, if any, is thought to be very low. Hormone producing ovarian tumors increase the risk as well. As related to hormones, obesity plays a role, actually reducing the risk in premenopausal patients (thought to be related to cycles in which there is no ovulation (anovulatory) and lower late cycle progesterone levels), and increasing the risk in postmenopausal patients (due to production of estrogens in the peripheral fat).

Environmental factors can contribute. Even apart from obesity, dietary factors have been implicated. A diet high in fats is thought to contribute, as does moderate to heavy alcohol consumption. Coffee intake has not been linked to breast cancer, and in spite of established links to many cancers, smoking has not been found to contribute to the risk for cancer of the breast. Other environmental factors include radiation exposure, such as following treatment for a previous cancer on the chest wall or in the middle section of the chest cavity (mediastinum).

Comparing geographic influences, an increased incidence is seen in United States and Western countries when compared to non-Western countries, with the risk for the US/Western group 4–7 times that of the non-Westerners. However, the non-Western risk has been shown to increase to levels seen in the Westerners over generations with relocation to those areas.

In the course of diagnosis, the usual clinical scenario is a woman who palpates a lump during self-examination of the breast. The woman is most often post-menopausal, although as mentioned earlier premenopausal cancers do occur. There are multiple types of biopsies and methods of diagnosis used to diagnose breast cancer, depending on the clinician and institution. For example, definitive diagnosis may consist of a mammogram, followed by a stereotactic guided needle biopsy. This type of biopsy utilizes mammogram and a computer program to assist the radiologist in determining the exact coordinates of the lesion, thereby aiding in placement of the needle. Often, the location is determined by the presence of microcalcifications, with linear microcalcifications being the most suspicious for malignancy (cancer, along with microcalcification tends to follow the duct structure). An X-ray is often taken of the biopsy material, to insure that the calcification is indeed present in the biopsy. A titanium clip is often placed in the breast at the biopsy site, in order to aid the surgeon in removal of the proper site, should the biopsy prove malignant and additional treatment be necessary.

Deciphering the Pathology Report

The pathology report aims to present factors that are known (and sometimes only suspected) to be important for determining prognosis, risk of recurrence, survival, and treatment. The most important factors are related to lymph node metastasis (greater than or equal to four positive nodes increasing the stage and worsening the prognosis), tumor size (greater than 2.0 cm being worse), histological grade (the higher the grade, the worse the prognosis – see below), presence of vascular/lymphatic invasion (worse if present), presence of hormone receptors (estrogen and progesterone receptor positivity tend to correlate with less aggressive tumors and also have implications for treatment options), and margin status (worse if positive margins).

Many other factors suspected to be important for prognosis have been and are being studied. Among these, Her2/neu, a gene which produces an epithelial growth factor-like protein (overexpression correlates with tumor aggressiveness, but has implications for treatment), DNA ploidy (aneuploid tumors correlate to higher grade), proliferation markers such as Ki-67 (higher percentage of cells proliferating or in S-phase correlates to more aggressive tumors), p53 (a tumor suppressor gene which when mutated tends to produce a defective protein thereby reducing the suppressive capacity), and a host of lesser studied factors.

The most used method currently for determining histological grade is based on the modification of the Bloom and Richardson grading system by Elston and Ellis (The Nottingham combined histologic grade, see chapter 7, table 7.1). This method takes into consideration three factors, with a possible score of 1–3 on each factor (Fig. 5.1). Histologic grade of invasive breast carcinoma has been shown to have strong association with long-term survival [6, 7].

The features of invasive ductal carcinoma that should be included in the final pathology report are listed in Table 5.1.

Table 5.1 Important features
of invasive ductal carcinoma
included in pathology report

Tumor size
Tumor margin
Tumor type
Tumor grade
Lymph node status if applicable
Lymphovascular invasion
Expression of biomarkers including:
ER
PR
Ki-67
Her-2/neu
DNA ploidy

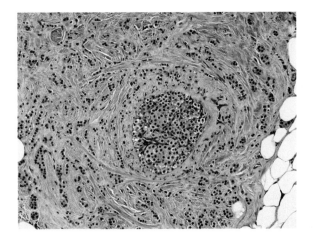

Fig. 5.2 Invasive lobular carcinoma. Tumor cells are small and discohesive, grow in a linear or single file pattern.

Invasive Lobular Carcinoma

Invasive lobular carcinoma is recognized as a malignancy so named because the similarity in appearance of the tumor cells with those seen in lobules. These neoplastic epithelial cells also invade the surrounding stroma in a characteristic fashion, usually distinct from the invasive ductal type. The patterns of invasion include linear rows of one or two cells wide, nests and diffuse, with a fibrotic (known as "desmoplastic") reaction of the stroma, see Fig. 5.2. This fibrotic stromal reaction is what makes some tumors feel firm or hard on palpation. The tumor cells are characteristically small and show little variation in size and appearance. Some cells show intracytoplasmic lumens which cause the nucleus to be displaced to one side, causing the microscopic appearance of "signet ring" cells. Tumors with greater than 10% signet ring cells have been shown to carry a worse overall prognosis. Invasive lobular carcinoma is known for its tendency to be accompanied by other lobular neoplasias (see Chap. 4), with some authors stating as many as

90% of cases having co-existent lobular carcinoma in situ and/or atypical lobular hyperplasia in the same or opposite breast. The presence of lobular carcinoma, both in situ and invasive, increases the risk of some type of carcinoma in the opposite breast (most but not all are lobular type). The lobular neoplasias also have a greater tendency to be present in more than one quadrant of the breast (multicentric), with up to 30% showing more than one focus of involvement.

The incidence of invasive lobular carcinoma ranges from 0.7 to 15% of invasive breast carcinomas, with the wide range being attributed to the differences in histological criteria by different investigators, as well as the more recent inclusion of several variant of histological patterns which were not included in earlier reports.

Clinical Presentation

The diffuse pattern of infiltration tends to make invasive lobular carcinoma more elusive both radiographically and by palpation than typical ductal carcinoma. Lobular carcinoma is known to present in heterogeneous patterns on imaging. Some are seen as asymmetric and ill-defined densities, with others appearing as only a thickening of the tissue. The tumors can vary from tiny to very large, and may even present with multiple small palpable nodules. Lobular carcinoma has a higher frequency of involving both breasts than ductal carcinoma. Furthermore, lobular carcinoma is less likely to be associated with microcalcifications than ductal carcinoma. These characteristics contribute to the mammographic problems sometimes encountered in diagnosis of lobular carcinoma.

Lobular carcinoma tends to be a disease of women beyond child-bearing age, with the median age being 45–57 years. However, lobular carcinoma has been diagnosed in younger women, with the age of presentation ranging from 26 to 86 years. The disease constitutes 11% of breast carcinomas in women over 75 years of age, but only 2% in those younger than 35. The range of bilateral tumors is 6–47% – and once diagnosed with invasive lobular carcinoma, the risk of having a tumor in the opposite breast is around 20%.

Several subtypes have been described for invasive lobular carcinoma, based on pattern of growth, cellular variation, or behavior. The most frequent is the "classic" pattern which is the linear or single file pattern. Another subtype is the "alveolar" type, in which neoplastic cells invade as nests and islands of 20 or more cells, and the "solid" type, which shows closely packed small cells forming large nests or sheets. Other variants include the so-called "mixed" pattern, where more than one architectural pattern is displayed, and tubulolobular pattern where tubule formation is seen co-existing with the single-file infiltrative pattern. Reports vary as to the prognostic differences between classic type and these variants, with some reports stating that the classic type has a better overall survival, while others reveal no significant difference. On the other hand, there is little disagreement about the "pleomorphic" pattern. This subtype carries the most ominous prognosis, with a known reduction in overall survival compared to classic (with less than 10% signet ring cells) and other variant lobular carcinomas, as well as ductal carcinomas.

Pleomorphic lobular carcinoma are cytologically more atypical with prominent nuclear pleomorphism.

Most studies show similar survival data for classic invasive lobular and invasive ductal carcinoma of no special type. This survival is intermediate between the less aggressive subtypes of ductal carcinoma (such as tubular carcinoma), and pleomorphic lobular and signet ring cell carcinomas, which have been shown to have a worse overall survival. Treatment is also similar with emphasis on breast conserving measures, despite the frequent multicentricity of lobular carcinoma.

Risk Factors and Diagnosis

The risk factors for invasive lobular carcinoma are similar to that for typical ductal types (see above) and include family history, presence of proliferative breast disease, and genetic and socioeconomic factors among others (see discussion under ductal carcinoma).

The diagnosis is often made by needle core biopsy, following an abnormal mammogram, sonogram, or discovery of a mass or thickened area by palpation.

Deciphering the Pathology Report

Important features that should be included in the pathology report are the same as discussed above for invasive ductal carcinoma, see Table 5.1. The grading system used for ductal carcinoma is also used for lobular types. However, since invasive lobular carcinoma cells are known to lack the cellular adhesion protein E-cadherin, a pathology report might also mention the presence or absence of this stain to differentiate lobular carcinoma from ductal carcinoma in questionable cases [8].

Lobular carcinoma is also less likely to express other surface markers when compared to invasive ductal carcinoma, including, Her2/neu and vascular endothelial growth factor.

Breast Cancer: The Special Types

Terminology, Clinical Presentation and Implications for Management

There are special types of breast carcinoma with distinct histologic and clinical features that worth separate discussions as following.

Tubular carcinoma is composed of distinct well-differentiated tubular structures with open lumina lined by a single layer of epithelial cells (Fig. 5.3). To qualify for

Fig. 5.3 Invasive tubular carcinoma. Tumor cells have low nuclear grade, and more than 90% of the tumor cells form tubular structures with open lumens.

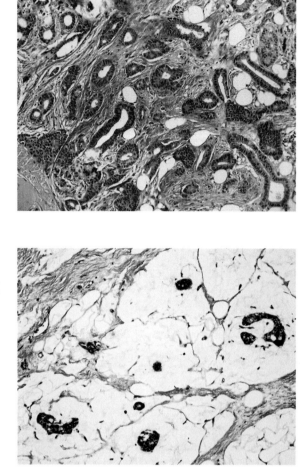

Fig. 5.4 Mucinous carcinoma. Clusters of small and uniform tumor cells float in a large quantity of extracellular mucin.

this diagnosis, 90% of the tumor should contain tubular structures. Pure tubular carcinomas are rare when strict criteria are applied to the diagnosis. In general, tubular carcinomas occur in older patients, are smaller in size and have less nodal metastasis. Tubular carcinomas have a particularly favorable prognosis compared to invasive carcinomas of no special type. They are almost always estrogen and progesterone receptor positive, have low proliferative activity, and are negative for Her-2/neu and epidermal growth factor receptor.

Mucinous carcinoma (colloid carcinoma) is characterized by clusters of small and uniform tumor cells floating in a large quantity of extracellular mucin (Fig. 5.4). It accounts for about 2% of all breast carcinomas and occurs in an older age group. Mammogram usually shows a well-circumscribed lobulated lesion. Grossly, it is soft with a gelatinous and glistening cut surface. Mucinous carcinoma is typically estrogen receptor and progesterone receptor positive. Pure mucinous carcinoma has an excellent prognosis with a 10-year survival ranging from 80 to 100%.

Fig. 5.5 Medullary carcinoma. Tumor cells grow in a syncytial pattern (no gland or tubule formation) with a prominent lymphoplasmacytic background.

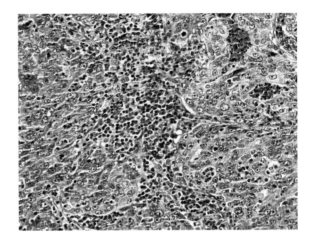

Medullary carcinoma is a well-circumscribed carcinoma with pushing margins. The tumor is composed of syncytial sheets of poorly differentiated large pleomorphic cells, with no glandular or tubular structures. Diffuse lymphoplasmcytic infiltrate in the tumor stroma is a prominent feature (Fig. 5.5). Complete histological circumscription is also a rule. Most medullary carcinomas are aneuploid with high proliferative activity. They typically lack estrogen receptors and progesterone receptors and have a low incidence of Her-2/neu overexpression [9]. Medullary carcinomas have a better prognosis than the usual invasive ductal carcinomas despite their poorly differentiated morphology. However, stringent diagnostic criteria should be followed to preserve this unique histological clinical identity of medullary carcinoma.

Invasive papillary carcinoma accounts for less than 2% of invasive breast carcinomas and carries a relatively good prognosis. It is typically well delineated, shows delicate or blunt papillae with focal solid areas of tumor growth. Most tumors are intermediate grade, positive for estrogen receptor and progesterone receptor, and negative for Her-2/neu overexpression.

Apocrine carcinoma is a carcinoma showing cytological features of apocrine cells in more than 90% of the tumor cells. It does not have distinct clinical features. The tumor cells are typically negative for estrogen receptor and progesterone receptor, and interestingly, express androgen receptors.

Metaplastic carcinoma refers to a heterogeneous group of tumors containing squamous cells and/or spindle cells with or without mesenchymal (stromal) differentiation. The metaplastic squamous or spindle cells may be the pure component of the tumor, or they may admix with a recognizable adenocarcinoma component. It accounts for less than 1% of all invasive mammary carcinoma. Clinically, it may present as a large (median size 3–4 cm) firm palpable mass. Thorough histologic sampling is necessary to identify different components, including squamous, glandular, spindle cell, chondroid or even osseous components. Metaplastic carcinomas in general are aggressive tumors with frequent axillary node metastases. Both the epithelial and mesenchymal components are negative for estrogen receptor and progesterone receptor. Currently, there is no efficient therapy for the management of metaplastic carcinoma.

Deciphering the Pathology Report

The pathology diagnosis should follow strict criteria for these special types of invasive breast cancers (the term carcinoma is cancer of epithelial origin and will be the term used in pathology reports) as they have distinct clinical significance. Pathology reports, in all cases, should specify the tumor type as follows:

- Invasive breast carcinoma, special type (specify)
- Invasive ductal carcinoma, NOS (not otherwise specified)
- Invasive lobular carcinoma, specify pattern (classic, solid, alveolar, and pleomorphic)
- Invasive mixed ductal and lobular carcinoma

The same details should be included in the report as discussed above for invasive ductal carcinoma.

References

1. Bradbury AR, Olopade OI (2007) Genetic susceptibility to breast cancer. Rev Endocr Metab Disord 8:225–267
2. Lester SC (2009) The breast. In: Kumar V, Abbas A et al (eds) Pathologic basis of disease, 8th ed. Saunders, Philadelphia, pp 1077–1078
3. Hayanga AJ, Newman LA (2007) Investigating the phenotypes and genotypes of breast cancer in women with African ancestry: the need for more genetic epidemiology. Surg Clin North Am 87:551–568
4. John EM et al (2007) Prevalence of pathogenic BRCA1 mutation carriers in 5 US racial/ethnic groups. JAMA 2007 298:2869–2876
5. Yager JD, Davidson NE (2006) Estrogen carcinogenesis in breast cancer. N Engl J Med 354:270–282
6. Elston CW, Ellis IO (1991) Pathological prognostic factors in breast cancer. I. The value of histological grade in breast cancer: experience from a large study with long-term follow-up. Histopathology 19:403–410
7. Page DL, Ellis IO, Elston CW (1995) Histologic grading of breast cancer. Let's do it. Am J Clin Pathol 103:123–124
8. Moll R, Mitze M, Frixen UH et al (1993) Differential loss of E-cadherin expression in infiltrating ductal and lobular breast carcinomas. Am J Pathol 143:1731–1742
9. Ellis IO, Schnitt SJ, Sastre-Garau X et al. (2003) Invasive breast carcinoma. In: Tavassoli FA, Devilee P (eds) World Health Organization of tumors, pathology and genetics: tumors of the breast and female genital organs. IARC Press, Lyon, pp 28–29

Chapter 6
Things Pathologists Must Always Consider

Joan Cangiarella

Keywords Fine needle aspiration • Core needle biopsy • Mimics of malignancy • Fibromatosis (f) • Granular cell tumor (f) • Granulomatous mastitis (f) • Fat necrosis (f) • Radial scar (f) • Core needle biopsy pitfalls • Nipple retracton • Pathology report • Frozen section • Nottingham–Bloom–Richardson • Margins • TNM • Fine needle aspiration biopsy

Mimics of Malignancy

Mimics of malignancy are usually rare lesions, but they merit discussion and represent something that pathologists always think about.

Fibromatosis

Fibromatosis occurs in women in the third to fourth decades of life. The significance of this lesion is that it may mimic cancer clinically (by physical examination) and radiographically. Fibromatosis usually grows slowly, is locally aggressive with the tendency to recur or reappear, but not metastasize. The cause remains unknown [1]. Fibromatosis presents as a palpable hard or firm mass, which may cause skin and nipple retraction creating a suspicion of malignancy [2]. Radiographically, fibromatosis may appear to be cancer because of its irregular shape, high density, and often spiculate appearance on mammogram (see Fig. 6.1) and its hypoechoic appearance with posterior acoustic shadowing on ultrasound [3]. Microscopically, fibromatosis is composed of a dense collagenous matrix with spindle-shaped cells. Often an infiltrative pattern into the surrounding fat is observed, leading to suspicion of malignancy. Wide local excision

J. Cangiarella (✉)
Associate Professor, Department of Pathology, New York University School of Medicine, New York, NY, USA
e-mail: joan.cangiarella@nymc.org

P.A. Thomas (ed.), *Breast Cancer and its Precursor Lesions*, Current Clinical Pathology, DOI 10.1007/978-1-60327-154-7_6, © Springer Science+Business Media, LLC 2011

Fig. 6.1 Fibromatosis: mammogram of the right breast shows an oval mass (*arrow*) with indistinct margins in the medial aspect.

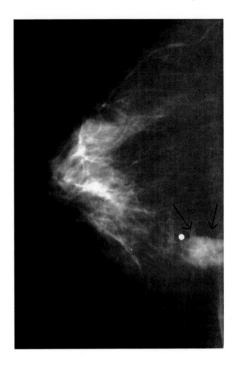

is the treatment of choice with re-excision if present at a margin. Recurrence rates at 10 years range from 24 to 77% [4]. Radiation, chemotherapy, or anti-estrogen therapy have all shown some effect in controlling the process.

Fat Necrosis

Fat necrosis of the breast is a benign inflammatory lesion. Trauma is the cause in the majority of cases; however, fat necrosis can be due to a host of other things, including biopsy, lumpectomy and radiation. Fat necrosis presents as a single mass, multiple round nodules, or less often as fixed irregular masses with retraction of overlying skin [5]. Mammographically, fat necrosis appears as lipid cysts, microcalcification, spiculate areas of increased opacity, and discrete masses [5]. Whereas some mammographic features of fat necrosis are characteristic such as well-defined lucency and peripheral rim calcification; other features are nonspecific, and malignancy must be excluded. Uncommonly fat necrosis presents as suspicious microcalcifications, simulating DCIS [6]. Fat necrosis may be seen as an ill-defined or spiculated lesion, just as cancer can appear [5]. Thus, new masses in patients following lumpectomy and radiation therapy must be evaluated to exclude recurrence of cancer [7]. On ultrasound, the findings vary, but can appear as solid masses [8] (see Fig. 6.2). To the unaided eye, fat necrosis may have the previously described spiculated appearance, similar to what is seen by mammogram. Microscopically, foamy, fat-filled macrophages and foreign body giant cells are seen in a background of chronic inflammation.

Fig. 6.2 Fat Necrosis: ultrasound of the right breast shows a complex cystic mass with posterior acoustic shadowing.

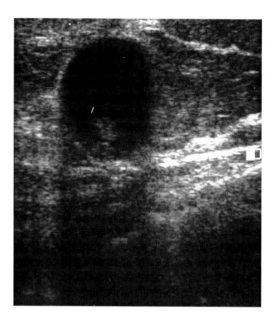

Granulomatous Mastitis

Granulomatous mastitis is an inflammatory disease of unknown cause. It primarily affects women shortly after childbirth and the clinical and mammographic findings often mimic those of cancer. The symptoms may include galactorrhea (spontaneous flow of milk from the breast not associated with pregnancy or lactation), inflammation, and/or mass with induration or ulceration of overlying skin [9]. On mammogram asymmetrical dense lesions, well-circumscribed opacities and spiculated lesions can be seen [10]. By ultrasound one sees an irregular mass with angulated borders (see Fig. 6.3). However, radiologic techniques including mammography, ultrasonography and magnetic resonance imaging (MRI) are not helpful in unequivocally distinguishing this entity from malignancy [11]. An accurate diagnosis is made by biopsy, wherein granulomatous inflammation with giant cells, macrophages and abscesses can be seen. Fine needle aspiration biopsy may be difficult, and cases of granulomatous mastitis have inadvertently been reported as malignant [10]. Other causes of granulomatous inflammation such as tuberculosis, sarcoidosis, and plasma cell mastitis must be excluded. Treatment includes excision with or without corticosteroid therapy [12].

Radial Scar

Radial scar (see also Chap. 3) is a benign proliferative lesion of the breast that may be confused mammographically with an invasive cancer, appearing again as a spiculated mass (see Fig. 6.4). Microscopically, a radial scar has a central fibrotic or

Fig. 6.3 Granulomatous
mastitis: ultrasound of the
left breast shows an irregular
shaped hypoechoic mass with
angulated margins.

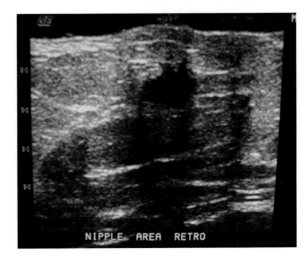

Fig. 6.4 Radial Scar:
mammogram of the left
breast shows an area of architectural distortion (*arrow*) in
the upper outer quadrant.

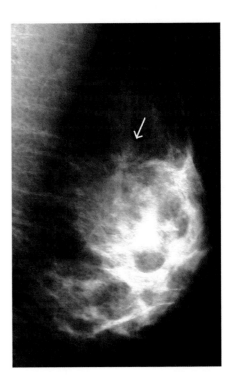

elastotic area with entrapped ducts and a surrounding proliferation of ducts and
lobules. The cause of radial scars is unknown, however, there is accumulating
evidence of an association with atypia and malignancy [13]. Fat can be trapped in
the center of the lesion causing lucency on mammogram and if present is a feature

that is helpful in distinguishing the radial scar from cancer. Microscopically, the major differential diagnosis is a special type of breast cancer called tubular carcinoma. However, the epithelium in tubular carcinoma lacks the second cell or myoepithelial cell layer classically present around the ducts of radial scars. Staining the tissue with markers for smooth muscle actin, calponin or p63, highlight the myoepithelial cells. Based on the results of studies showing an increased risk of finding concomitant carcinoma in large radial scars, excision is recommended [14].

Granular Cell Tumor

Granular cell tumor is a tumor is usually seen in women between 30 and 50 years and is more common in premenopausal African American women [15]. This lesion is particularly difficult to diagnose correctly preoperatively as the clinical signs, mammographic, ultrasonographic, and pathologic findings often suggest carcinoma [16]. Granular cell tumors grow slowly and are often firm, painless, and poorly marginated [16]. When superficial, a granular cell tumor can cause retraction of the skin mimicking cancer. The mammographic findings are variable and can present as round, circumscribed masses, indistinct densities, or as a spiculated mass indistinguishable from carcinoma, see Figure 6.5. Ultrasound may also show solid masses with irregular margins and marked posterior shadowing, as seen in carcinoma [17]. On examination with the un-aided eye, these tumors usually feel firm, and look gray-white or yellow. Even under the microscope, this tumor due to its irregular edges may simulate carcinoma. Microscopically, nests and sheets of cells with abundant granular cytoplasm and small central nuclei are seen. S-100 protein cytoplasmic staining of the granular cells is indicative of origin from Schwannian cells of peripheral nerves. The treatment of a granular cell tumor is wide excision. Most granular cell tumors are benign, but malignant granular cell tumors have been reported [18].

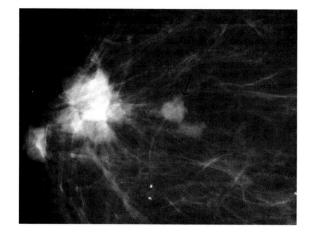

Fig. 6.5 Granular cell tumor: mammogram of the right breast shows one large spiculate mass (*thick arrow*) and adjacent small irregular mass in the periareolar region.

What Should Always Be in Any Pathology Report?

The Pathology Report

The pathology report is a very important document and the information written in it will determine treatment and predict outcome and it is therefore very important that non-pathologists have an unequivocal understanding of the information in the report; but, patients are also major stakeholders and should be empowered to understand the information that the report is conveying. What follows are general components, Chap. 6 details components of a report for breast cancer, but some of these components may vary by institution.

The pathology report is assigned a unique identifying number for each patient. The report should always have patient information, including name, date of birth, gender, date of surgery. The report includes a "gross" or macroscopic description of what the tissue looks like when examined by the pathologist with their un-aided eye. The macroscopic description includes the type of specimen received (a needle core biopsy, a lumpectomy, a segmental excision or a mastectomy). Masses or cysts are described noting their color, size, and shape with an evaluation of the margins of the sample. Size may not be able to be determined by the pathologist if it was biopsied by core needle or fine needle aspiration biopsy. If lymph nodes were removed, number and size must be reported. If the lesion appears malignant to the unaided eye or is a known malignancy, very careful evaluation of the margins with a statement of how close the tumor is to the edge of the specimen is given. The specimen should be "oriented"(arranged the way it was located anatomically in the breast). This information is important as it guides the surgeon to the area of concern in the breast if a margin was positive and re-excision was necessary. Definitive information about the margin is usually obtained at microscopic examination. If a frozen section (a pathologist's microscopic evaluation of portion of the tumor or sentinel lymph node during the operation) was performed, this should be mentioned in the report, as well as their rapid preliminary diagnosis. The frozen section diagnosis is not the final diagnosis. The final diagnosis is a section of its own within the pathology report and is made after the specimen has been more completely sampled, processed appropriately and thoroughly examined by the pathologist. In a small number of cases the frozen section rapid diagnosis is not the same as the final diagnosis. Usually, such discrepancies, while rare, do not alter the management of the patient.

Reports variably include a "microscopic" description of the features of the tissue when examined under the microscope. The microscopic description characterizes the tumor and all the features observed that lead to the final diagnosis. The pathology report will indicate the grade of the tumor, whether a separate section for microscopic description is included or not. The grade is based on the degree of differentiation; low grade tumor cells appear most similar to the normal cell of origin of the tumor and thus are well-differentiated. High grade tumor cells vary widely in their size and shapes and appear less like their cell of origin making them poorly differentiated. Moderately differentiated tumors are in the middle. Various grading schemes are used to classify tumors, but the Nottingham–Bloom–Richardson system is widely used [19]. The details of this grading system can be found in Chap. 7.

A statement regarding margins is usually included in the report. Margin, in this instance, refers to the distance between the tumor cells and the edge of the tissue. If the margin is free of tumor then additional surgery most likely will not be necessary. Tumors that are at the margin or close to the surgical margin (usually indicated by a measurement of how close) will most likely require reoperation to obtain a clear margin. The presence of tumor within the lymphatic spaces or within blood vessels should be noted as this usually is associated with a poorer outcome.

The pathology report must describe the number of lymph nodes actually identified microscopically. This number could differ from the number described in the macroscopic portion of the report. It should be stated whether or not tumor was identified in them and how many of the lymph nodes had cancer as well as the number that did not. The location and the size of the cancer in the nodes should also be described. This is critical for staging.

The report will include the pathological stage of the tumor. The American Joint Committee for Cancer (AJCC) manual for staging of Cancer uses the TNM classification system. The TNM system takes into consideration three components; T for tumor size, N for presence or absence of regional lymph node metastasis and M for the presence or absence of distant metastasis. The pathologic stage includes the size of the tumor and the presence or absence of regional lymph node metastases, i.e. the extent of the tumor or how much tumor is identified. Additional tests, other biopsies and/or imaging studies, may be necessary to determine if the tumor has spread to sites away from the areas near the breast to establish the final stage. Stage correlates with a patient's outcome or potential behavior of the tumor.

Finally, the pathology report may contain a "comment" section. Important information is often conveyed within this section. Information about special stains or procedures performed may be located in this section as well as anything unusual or distinguishing about the diagnosis. This section may include information about how this diagnosis compares to a previous one for the same patient. Sometimes a diagnosis maybe rare or not obvious, and a discussion of why this is the case and the possible diagnoses to be considered will be the in this section. This section may also contain recommendations for further testing to aid in arriving at the accurate diagnosis.

The College of American Pathologists (CAP) is the largest association composed of pathologists exclusively and as a dedicated advocate for patients and high quality care created a very useful and patient friendly cancer information website, MyBiopsy.org that also discusses how to read pathology reports. MyBiopsy.org provides information on breast and 39 other cancers as well as survivor stories, as well as access to a link that helps patients schedule cancer screening tests.

What Are the Limitations of Biopsy Techniques?

Core Needle Biopsy

Core needle biopsy obtains cylinders of breast tissue for microscopic analysis. This allows pathologists to see patterns and location of tumor cells, and thus make more specific diagnoses. Core biopsy can also provide assessment of invasiveness of a tumor, and analysis of biomarkers, characteristics that may influence particular treatment strategies. The diagnosis of most tumors on core biopsy is straightforward, but some lesions are difficult to evaluate accurately by core biopsy and lead to dilemmas regarding appropriate clinical management.

The reported sensitivity of core needle biopsy for the detection of malignancy ranges from 86 to 97% [20–23]. One disadvantage of core biopsy is the underestimation of carcinoma. A diagnosis of atypia on core biopsy still requires excision as underestimation of carcinoma in seen in 20–56% of cases with automated 14 gauge core needle and in 0–38% of cases in reports of vacuum assisted core needle biopsy [24].

Another disadvantage of core needle biopsy is that it samples part of a mass and invasive foci are often missed. For example, cases diagnosed as intraductal adenocarcinoma on core needle biopsy (non-invasive) may be upstaged to invasive carcinoma at excision in 16–35% of cases with automated 14 gauge core needle biopsy and from 0 to 19% of cases with vacuum assisted biopsy [24].

Certain lesions pose difficulty with regard to management when diagnosed at core biopsy. For example, LCIS on core biopsy is associated with invasive carcinoma in 25% of cases at excision [25]. Papillary lesions may appear benign on core biopsy but are upstaged to carcinomas in 5% of cases at excision [26]. Some of the factors that are associated with upgrading on excision are seen in Table 6.1. Unusual or uncommon lesions on core biopsy require a cautious and conservative approach. Distinguishing mucinous carcinoma from benign mucinous lesions can be difficult on core biopsy.

Core needle biopsy may completely remove or obscure a mammographic lesion, thus placement of a localizing metallic clip at the time of biopsy is mandatory to allow accurate localization if excision is necessary.

Table 6.1 Factors associated with subsequent upgrading a core needle biopsy diagnosis on excision

- Number of atypical epithelial foci (>2)
- Presence of micropapillary architecture
- Incomplete removal of the lesion
- Microcalcifications

Provenzano E, Pinder SE (2009) Pre-operative diagnosis of breast cancer in screening: problems and pitfalls. Pathology 41(1):3–17

What Are the Limitations of Fine Needle Aspiration Biopsy?

Fine needle aspiration biopsy is a diagnostic technique that involves the insertion of thin needles (22–27 gauge) into a breast lesion to obtain cells for diagnosis. This procedure can be done by palpation if the lesion can be felt or with the use of radiologic imaging such as mammography, ultrasound or MRI when lesions cannot be felt. The advantages of this technique is that it is a rapid, accurate, and cost-effective when performed by trained skilled operators and interpreted by pathologists with experience in this method. Some studies comparing fine needle aspiration with core biopsy prefer core biopsy due to the claim of fewer false negatives and inadequate and atypical diagnoses and most pathologists are more comfortable with samples of tissue compared to cytologic samples (which require specialty training for interpretation) thus, they feel core biopsies lead to more specific diagnoses. The disadvantage of this technique is that since only cells are obtained, the extent of invasiveness of a tumor cannot be made reliable. The presence of invasion obviously is important as the treatment differs between non-invasive (or in situ) cancer and invasive ones. One study demonstrated that 98% of palpable tumors diagnosed as cancer are invasive, but many surgeons prefer a tissue biopsy which is 99% reliable [27]. Other disadvantages of aspiration biopsy include unacceptably high inadequacy rate of fine needle aspiration seen in many institutions and the fact that it requires a level of cytopathology expertise not be available in all institutions.

The level of accuracy for fine needle aspiration ranges from 62 to 89% [28]. Aspiration biopsy however does replace surgery in many benign conditions. The use of FNA in the diagnosis of cancer of the breast has diminished as core biopsies have become standard at many institutions.

References

1. Rosen PP, Ernsberger D (1989). Mammary fibromatosis: a benign spindle-cell tumor with significant risk for local recurrence. Cancer 63:1363–1369
2. Schwarz GS, Drotman M, Rosenblatt R, Milner L et al (2006) Fibromatosis of the breast: case report and current concepts in the management of an uncommon lesion. Breast J 12:66–71
3. Mesurolle B, Ariche-Cohen M, Mignon F, Piron D, Guomot P-A (2001) Unusual mammographic and ultrasonography findings in fibromatosis of the breast. Eur Radiol 11:2241–2243
4. Gronchi A, Casal PG, Mariani L et al (2003) Quality of surgery and outcome in extra-abdominal aggressive fibromatosis: a series of patients surgically treated at a single institution. J Clin Oncol 21:1390–1397
5. Hogge JP, Robinson RE, Magnant CM, Zuurbier RA (1995) The mammographic spectrum of fat necrosis of the breast. Radiographics 15:1347–1356
6. Hogge JP, Hayes CW, Martin P (1995) Traumatic fat necrosis simulating intraductal carcinoma: a case report. Appl Radiol 24:37–38
7. Boyages J, Bilous M, Barraclough B, Langlands AO (1988) Fat necrosis of the breast following lumpectomy and radiation therapy for early breast cancer. Radiother Oncol 13:69–74
8. Bilgen IG, Ustun EE, Memis A (2001) Fat necrosis of the breast: clinical, mammographic and sonographic features. Eur J Radiol 39:92–99

9. Diesing D, Axt-Fliedner R, Hornung D, Weiss JM, Diedrich K, Friedrich M (2004) Granulomatous mastitis. Arch Gynecol Obstet 269:233–236

10. Bani-Hani KE, Yaghan RJ, Matalka II, Shatnawi NJ (2004) Idiopathic granulomatous mastitis: time to avoid unnecessary mastectomy. Breast J 10:318–322

11. Asoglu O, Ozmen V, Karanlik H et al (2005) Feasibility of surgical management in patients with granulomatous mastitis. Breast J 11:534–535

12. Imoto S, Kitaya T, Kodama T, Hasebe T, Mukai K (1997) Idiopathic granulomatous mastitis: case report and review of the literature. Jpn J Clin Oncol 27:274–277

13. Kennedy M, Masterson AV, Flanagan F (2003) Pathology and clinical relevance of radial scars: a review. J Clin Pathol 56:721–724

14. Sloane JP, Mayers MM (1993) Carcinoma and atypical hyperplasia in radial scars and complex sclerosing lesions: importance of lesion size and patient age. Histopathology 23:225–231

15. Gogas J, Markopoulos C, Kouskos E et al (2002) Granular cell tumor of the breast: a rare lesion resembling breast cancer. Eur J Gynaecol Oncol 23:333–334

16. Delaloye JF, Seraj F, Guillou L (2002) Granular cell tumor of the breast: a diagnostic pitfall. Breast 11:316–319

17. Adeniran A, Al-Ahmadie H, Mahoney MC, Robinson-Smith TM (2004) Granular cell tumor of the breast: a series of 17 cases and review of the literature. Breast J 10:528–531

18. Chetty R, Kalan MR (1992) Malignant granular cell tumor of the breast. J Surg Oncol 49:135–137

19. Elston CW, Ellis IO (1991) Pathological prognostic factors in breast cancer. I. The value of histological grade in breast cancer: experience from a large study with long-term follow-up. Histopathology 19:403–410

20. Westenend PJ, Sever AR, Beekman-de Volder HJC et al (2001) A comparison of aspiration cytology and core needle biopsy in the evaluation of breast lesions. Cancer 93:146–150

21. Hatada T, Ishii H, Ichii S et al (2000) Diagnostic value of ultrasound-guided fine-needle aspiration biopsy, core needle biopsy, and evaluation of combined use in the diagnosis of breast lesions. J Am Coll Surg 190:299–303

22. Ballo MS, Sneige N (1996) Can core needle biopsy replace fine-needle aspiration cytology in the diagnosis of palpable breast carcinoma. A comparative study of 124 women. Cancer 78:773–777

23. Oyama T, Koibuchi Y, McKee G (2004) Core needle biopsy (CNB) as a diagnostic method for breast lesions: comparison with fine needle aspiration cytology (FNA). Breast Cancer 11:339–342

24. Liberman L (2000) Clinical management issues in percutaneous core breast biopsy. Radiol Clin North Am 38:791–807

25. Levine PH, Simsir A, Cangiarella J (2006) Management issues in breast lesions diagnosed by fine needle aspiration and percutaneous core breast biopsy. Am J Clin Pathol 125(suppl):S124–S134

26. Mercado CL, Hamele-Bena D, Oken SM, Singer CI, Cangiarella J (2006) Papillary lesions of the breast on percutaneous core biopsy. Radiology 238:801–808

27. Chhieng DC, Fernandez G, Cangiarella J et al (2000) Invasive carcinoma in clinically suspicious breast masses diagnosed as adenocarcinoma by fine-needle aspiration. Cancer 90:96–101

28. Pisano ED, Fajardo LL, Caudry JJ, Sneige N, Frable WJ, Berg WA, Tocino I, Schnitt SJ, Connolly JL, Gatsonis CA, McNeil BJ (2001) Fine-needle aspiration biopsy of non-palpable breast lesions in a multicenter clinical trial: results from the radiologic diagnostic oncology group V. Radiology 219:785–792

Chapter 7
Nuances and Details of the Pathology Report

Fang Fan

Keywords Prognostic markers (f) • Neoadjuvant therapy • Sentinel lymph node biopsy • Equivocal diagnoses • Microinvasive • p63 • Pagetoid spread • Lobular extension • Prognostic information • Marker panel (f) • Histologic grade • Lymph node status • Lymphovascular invasion • Perineural invasion • Paget's disease • Molecular markers • Fluorescent in situ hybridization • FISH • HercepTest • Molecular subtypes • Triple negative

Equivocal or Non-committal Diagnoses

On occasion, the pathologist may have insufficient tissue to make a diagnosis, the tissue is altered or damaged in processing, or lesions may have overlapping features, but the lesion was not sampled in a way to make a definitive diagnosis, i.e., core needle versus excision. In those instances, the pathology report is likely to contain language like "consistent with", "suggestive of", "favor" "cannot exclude". One should take note of such language and confer with your pathologist to determine what precisely the issues are and what information she or he is trying to convey. When these words are used, the pathologist may be thinking that they have "communicated" that the diagnosis is equivocal, but a non-pathologist may think otherwise. The best way to establish the most appropriate diagnosis is always using the "triple test", clinical/radiologic/pathologic correlation. If the diagnoses or terms in the pathology report are not consistent with either the clinical and/or radiologic exam, further investigation is warranted.

F. Fan (✉)
Associate Professor, Department of Pathology and Laboratory Medicine,
University of Kansas Medical Centre, Kansas City, KS, USA
e-mail: ffan@kumc.edu

P.A. Thomas (ed.), *Breast Cancer and its Precursor Lesions*, Current Clinical Pathology,   63
DOI 10.1007/978-1-60327-154-7_7, © Springer Science+Business Media, LLC 2011

In Situ vs. Microinvasive vs. Invasive Breast Carcinoma

There is no generally accepted agreement on the definition of microinvasive carcinoma. Most commonly, it is defined as the presence of one or more small microscopic foci of tumor (none exceeding 1 mm) infiltrating into the surrounding interlobular stroma in a background of ductal carcinoma in situ [1] (Fig. 7.1). Microinvasion is most often associated with periductal desmoplastic fibrosis or periductal/perilobular lymphocytic infiltrate, features of high-grade or comedo DCIS. When in doubt, deeper sections and immunohistochemical stains for myoepithelial cells, including smooth muscle myosin and p63, are helpful.

Microinvasive carcinoma remains to be an evolving area, needing a generally accepted definition and follow-up data. Currently, there are no specific clinical features associated with microinvasive breast carcinoma, and the condition is generally managed as it is for ductal carcinoma in situ. A pathology report for microinvasive carcinoma should provide the number of microinvasive foci and the size of the largest focus.

Lobular Extension/Pagetoid Spread

Ductal carcinoma in situ may invade through the basement membrane to the stroma, or spread within the ductal-lobular unit to involve the entire lobule. The latter is called lobular extension or cancerization of the lobule (Fig. 7.2). The way the tumor cells spread through the ductal system is called pagetoid spread (Fig. 7.3).

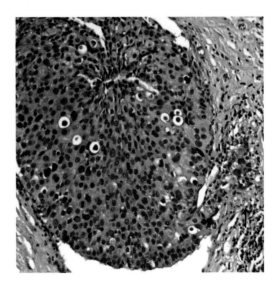

Fig. 7.1 Microinvasive breast carcinoma. A small microscopic focus of tumor cells invades through the basement membrane into the surrounding stroma (arrow). The invasive focus is less than 1 mm in size.

Fig. 7.2 Cancerization
of the lobule. The terminal
ductal lobular unit is
expanded and filled with
malignant cells spreading
from ductal carcinoma in situ.

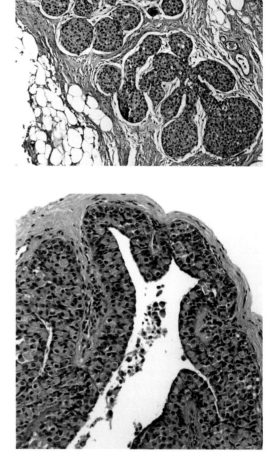

Fig. 7.3 Pagetoid spread of
tumor cells. Large tumor cells
are seen scattered in the wall
of the duct.

Prognostic Information That Can Be Obtained from the Pathology Report

Tumor Size

Tumor size is one of the most important prognostic factors a pathology report can provide because it decides the T (tumor) staging in the TNM staging of a tumor [2]. Unfortunately, there is a great variability in how pathologists record tumor size.

There is often poor correlation between the gross and microscopic measurement of tumor size. If a tumor is grossly visible, it is measured grossly and correlates later with the microscopic measurement. If no gross tumor is identified, the measurement is performed microscopically. When there is a discrepancy between the gross and microscopic size of the invasive tumor, the microscopic measurement should be used and indicated in the pathology report [3]. It is important to stress that only the size of invasive carcinoma should be used for the pathologic staging (pT), not a size that includes both invasive and in situ carcinomas. When multiple separate invasive tumor foci are present, the size should be recorded individually in the pathology report and only the largest focus is used for staging. It is not recommended to add different tumor sizes together.

Histologic Grade

Many studies have shown a significant association between histologic grade (how similar or dissimilar the tumor cells look compared to the normal cells) and survival in invasive breast carcinoma [4]. The currently well-adopted grading system is a modification by Elston and Ellis of the Bloom and Richardson system. It includes evaluation of three histologic features: nuclear pleomorphism, tubule and gland formation, and mitotic counts (Table 7.1). This grading scheme is recommended for all invasive carcinomas of the breast, regardless of morphological type. Histologic grade may also serve as a predictive factor with regard to response to

Table 7.1 Histologic grading of invasive breast carcinomas (from Elston and Ellis's modification of the Scarff–Bloom–Richardson method)

- Features evaluated:
- Tubule and gland formation
    1. Majority of tumor (>75%)
    2. Moderate degree (10–75%)
    3. Little or none (<10%)
- Nuclear pleomorphism
    1. Small, regular uniform cells
    2. Moderate increase in size and variability
    3. Marked variation
- Mitotic counts

Field diameter (mm)	0.44	0.59	0.63
Field area (mm^2)	0.152	0.274	0.312
1	0–5	0–9	0–11
2	6–10	10–19	12–22
3	>11	>20	>23

Final grade (combining values of the above three features):
Grade 1: Well differentiated, 3–5 points
Grade 2: Moderately differentiated, 6–7 points
Grade 3: Poorly differentiated, 8–9 points

chemotherapy in that high histological grade is associated with a better response to certain chemotherapy than low histological grade.

Lymph Node Status

Lymph node status is the single most important prognostic factor in breast cancer. As the number of positive nodes increases, disease free and overall survival rates decrease. Pathology reports should state clearly the number of positive lymph nodes as it denotes the N staging in the tumor TNM staging. The size of the largest tumor deposit in the positive lymph node, and the presence or absence of extranodal extension should also be recorded because it affects management decision.

Sentinel lymph node biopsy has become the standard of practice since early 1990s to replace the complete axillary lymph node dissection with low morbidity rate [5]. Although it is common for pathologists to use step sections and immunohistochemistry to evaluate sentinel lymph nodes, it is not a required recommendation.

Isolated tumor cells (ITCs) is defined as single cells or small clusters of cells <0.2 mm in size detected by immunohistochemistry or H&E-stained sections. The patient is staged as pN0 (i+). Micrometastasis is defined as tumor focus >0.2 mm but none >2.0 mm in the lymph node. The clinical significance of micrometastases and isolated tumor cells in the nodes, particularly those identified exclusively by immunohistochemistry, remains a matter of debate.

Lymphovascular Invasion

Lymphovascular invasion (LVI) has been shown to have an adverse effect on clinical outcome [6]. The major value of LVI is to identify patients with increased risk of axillary lymph node involvement. However, there is variability in pathologists to identify LVI. LVI must be distinguished from retraction artifacts of the stroma around tumor cell nests.

Perineural Invasion

Perineural invasion has not been shown to be an independent prognostic factor. It may be included in pathology reports if observed in the tumor.

Tumor Margins

When a breast excision specimen (lumpectomy or mastectomy) is received in pathology, the surgical excision margins (the outer surface of the specimen) are inked. A lumpectomy specimen is usually inked with different colors to indicate superior, inferior, anterior, posterior, medial and lateral margins; a mastectomy specimen is usually inked at its posterior surface to indicate the deep margin. The pathologist then examines the specimen grossly and microscopically to document the distance of tumor (invasive carcinoma and ductal carcinoma in-situ) to different margins. An adequate tumor clearance distance is important to ensure complete tumor removal and to decrease the local recurrence rate. Re-excision of positive or close margins may be necessary.

Extent of Ductal Carcinoma In Situ

Extensive ductal carcinoma in situ (comprising >25% of the lesion) occurring with invasive carcinoma is associated with high local recurrence in patients treated with breast conservation surgery and therefore should be noted in the pathology report.

Involvement of Skin and Nipple

Paget's disease of the nipple is seen in 1–4% of patients with breast cancer. It presents as an eczematous lesion in the area of nipple/areola. Histologic examination shows malignant glandular epithelial cells present singly or in clusters within epidermis (Fig. 7.4). The majority of Paget's disease (>95%) is associated with an underlying high-grade ductal carcinoma in situ with or without invasive carcinoma. Those associated with limited single duct involvement may be treated with breast conservation surgery; but most disease is often widespread. Very rarely, an underlying carcinoma cannot be found after extensive sampling; the disease may arise within the epidermis.

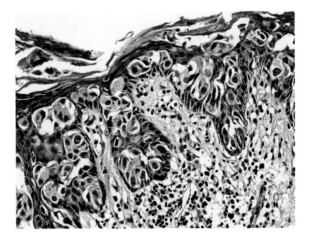

Fig. 7.4 Paget's disease of the nipple. Malignant epithelial cells are seen in the epidermis.

Fig. 7.5 Inflammatory breast carcinoma. There is extensive dermal lymphatic involvement by tumor cells.

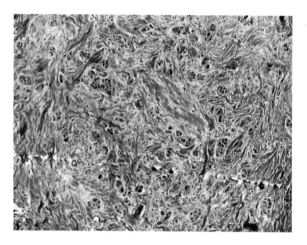

Paget's disease in itself does not have increased prognostic significance. It is staged as pTis-Paget's. Differential diagnoses include malignant melanoma and Bowen's disease. The distinctions can be made with immunohistochemical stains.

Sometimes, the breast skin presents with erythema, edema, warmth, tenderness, and puckering (so called "peau d'orange"), a breast skin biopsy shows extensive tumor emboli involving dermal lymphatic channels (Fig. 7.5). This form of locally advanced breast cancer is called "inflammatory carcinoma" and is staged clinically as T4d.

Molecular Markers in Breast Cancer

A panel of molecular markers is always performed on invasive breast carcinomas to guide therapy and predict prognosis. These include estrogen receptor (ER), progesterone receptor (PR), Her-2/neu, Ki-67 and p53. Nearly all markers are determined by standardized immunohistochemistry (IHC) assays in pathology laboratories with validated methods and strict quality control, see Fig. 7.6.

Estrogen/progesterone receptors (ER/PR) are nuclear transcription factors involved in breast development, growth, and differentiation. They are strong predictors of response to hormonal therapies, such as tamoxifen, other selective estrogen receptor modulators (SERM), and aromatase inhibitors [7]. About 70% of breast cancers are ER positive. The cut-off to define a positive ER varies; there is convincing data now to support that even 1% ER positive tumor respond to hormone therapy. Almost all well differentiated and most moderately differentiated breast cancers are positive for ER and PR.

Her-2/neu belongs to the human epidermal growth factor receptor family and is a transmembrane tyrosine kinase receptor that is involved in the regulatory pathways

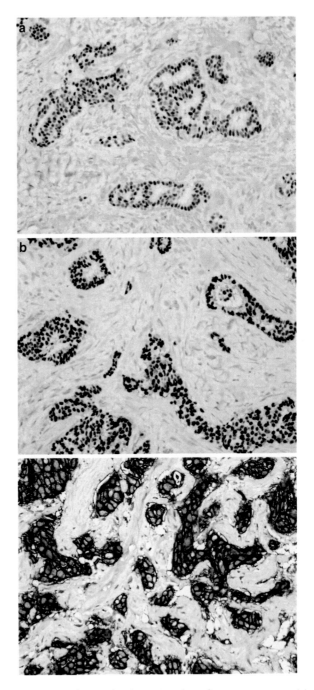

Fig. 7.6 Invasive breast carcinoma showing expression of estrogen receptor (**a**), progesterone receptor (**b**), and Her-2/neu (**c**).

of breast proliferation. Her-2/neu is associated with poor prognosis but predicts response to trastuzumab which targets the tyrosine kinase receptor [8].

The two commonly used methods to measure Her-2/neu are fluorescent in situ hybridization (FISH) for gene amplification and IHC for protein overexpression. The FDA approved tests are HercepTest for IHC and PathVysion for FISH. American Society of Clinical Oncology and College of American Pathologists have published guidelines stating that FISH results should be concordant with the corresponding IHC results in 95% of cases [9]. If both FISH and IHC are performed on the same tumor, the results should be correlated. In general, equivocal IHC results should be verified by FISH. When there is a major discrepancy between FISH and IHC results, the most common reason is that one of the assays is performed incorrectly; although there is a possibility of amplification without protein overexpression or protein overexpression without gene amplification in a small number of tumors. There is not a gold standard test in evaluating Her-2/neu. Laboratories perform Her-2/neu testing should follow rigorous quality control procedures and reporting guidelines and enroll in an external quality assurance program. It is hoped that the best approach to measure Her-2/neu in breast cancer will be established soon with the currently ongoing clinical trials and research.

Ki-67 is a marker of proliferative activity of cells and is detected by MIB-1 antibody. Tumors with high Ki-67 proliferation index behave more aggressively [10]. The cut-off to define a high proliferation index is not established.

p53 is a tumor suppressor gene that encodes a nuclear phosphoprotein involved in the regulation of cell cycle, DNA repair and apoptosis. In the lab, immunohistochemical stain detects mutated non-functional p53 protein in the tumor. About one third or more breast cancers have muted p53. Loss of p53 is associated with poor clinical outcome.

The pathology report or a separate addendum report may contain digital images of the panel of markers used, as well as the results, see Fig. 7.7.

Molecular Subtypes of Invasive Breast Cancer

Invasive breast carcinomas historically have been classified by the way they look, i.e., resemblance to a ductal cell or a lobular cell. Recent advances have provided new classification schemes based on their molecular markers (protein biomarkers) expression, such as luminal markers, ER/PR and Her-2/neu (Table 7.2). Such classification schemes promise to provide improved predictive (predict response to chemotherapy and selection of the most effective available chemotherapy) and prognostic (outcome, i.e., whether tumor will recur, metastasize to distant sites and/or overall survival) values [11]. The triple-negative (ER-/PR-/Her2-) or basal-like breast cancers do not respond to endocrine therapy or herceptin and have poor prognosis. Studies are ongoing to develop gene expression profiles that might further improve predictive and prognostic information. Gene profiles have been described that are associated with response to

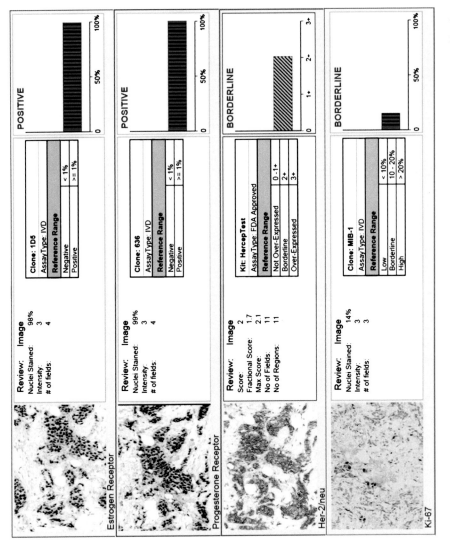

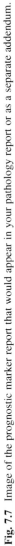

Fig. 7.7 Image of the prognostic marker report that would appear in your pathology report or as a separate addendum.

Table 7.2 Molecular subtypes of invasive breast cancer

	Luminal A	Luminal B	Her2/neu	Basal-like
ER	+	+	−	−
PR	+	+	−	−
Her2/neu	−	+	+	−
Clinical features	About 70% of breast cancers		About 15% of breast cancers	About 15% of breast cancers
	Respond to endocrine therapy		Respond to herceptin	No response to endocrine therapy or herceptin
	Relatively good prognosis			Relatively poor prognosis

chemotherapy (adjuvant and neoadjuvant), recurrence, distant metastasis, and even potential site of distant metastasis.

Clinical and Pathologic Stage

While histologic grade reflects tumor differentiation, tumor stage indicates the extent of disease. The AJCC (American Joint Committee on Cancer) cancer staging manual is used to stage breast cancer using the TNM system (T-tumor size, N-lymph node status, M-distant metastasis). Pathologic staging (pTNM) is performed after a therapeutic surgical procedure with the evaluation of tumor size and lymph node status on the excised specimens. Clinical staging is done based on clinical and radiological assessment of tumor size, lymph node status and the status of distant tumor metastasis. Clinicians use information from both the clinical stage and pathologic stage when evaluating an individual patient.

Neoadjuvant vs. Adjuvant Therapy and Pathologists' Role

Breast cancer was traditionally treated by surgical excision followed by adjuvant chemotherapy and/or radiation therapy. Neoadjuvant chemotherapy implies that the patient receives chemotherapy before the complete surgical removal of the carcinoma. One of the major benefits of neoadjuvant chemotherapy is that it reduces the size of large cancers, enabling the surgeon to remove the previously inoperable tumor or to excise the residual tumor by a more limited operation, such as lumpectomy instead of mastectomy. The response to neoadjuvant chemotherapy provides useful information about the potential response of the tumor to further treatment and in general may be informative about the biology of the carcinoma under treatment. Neoadjuvant chemotherapy is offered to patients with locally advanced breast caner and can also be offered as an alternative to adjuvant treatment to patients who are expected to receive chemotherapy for their cancers.

Assessment of the therapeutic response and measurement of residual disease in the breast and/or axillary lymph node is important because it may predict survival and provide guidelines for further therapy. Pathologic assessment of the final surgical resection specimen is the gold standard for determining a tumor's response to neoadjuvant chemotherapy [12]. When the tumor bed is extensively sampled and no residual invasive carcinoma is identified (DCIS may be present), this is termed complete pathologic response. When residual invasive carcinoma is identified along with features of therapy induced changes, this is called partial response. When invasive carcinoma remains the same size as prior to neoadjuvant chemotherapy with no therapy effect seen, this is categorized as no response. Pathologists examine the excised specimens systematically and thoroughly to document the presence or absence of residual tumor and treatment effects. The pathologic parameters that should be included in a pathology report after breast cancer neoadjuvant chemotherapy (if residual tumor is identified) include tumor type, size, grade, margins, and biomarkers (ER/PR/Her-2). Tumor staging after neoadjuvant chemotherapy should have a prefix of "y" as ypTNM to differentiate from the ones without neoadjuvant chemotherapy [13].

References

1. Schnitt SJ, Collins LC (2009) Microinvasive carcinoma. In: Biopsy interpretation of the breast. Lippincott Williams and Wilkins, Philadelphia, pp 236–248
2. AJCC (2010) Cancer staging handbook, 7th edn. Springer, New York
3. Lester SC, Bose S, Chen YY et al (2009) Protocol for the examination of specimens from patients with invasive carcinoma of the breast. Arch Pathol Lab Med 133:1515–1538
4. Rakha EA, El-Sayed ME, Lee AHS et al (2008) Prognostic significance of Nottingham histologic grade in invasive breast carcinoma. J Clin Oncol 26:3153–3158
5. Schwartz GF, Giuliano AE, UVeronesi2002Proceedings of the consensus conference on the role of sentinel lymph node biopsy in carcinoma of the breast, April 19–22, 2001, Philadelphia, Pennsylvania. Cancer 94:2542–2551
6. Mohammed RA, Martin SG, Gill MS et al (2007) Improved methods of detection of lymphovascular invasion demonstrate that it is the predominant method of vascular invasion in breast cancer and has important clinical consequences. Am J Surg Pathol 31:1825–1833
7. Harris L, Fritsche H, Mennel R et al (2007) American Society of Clinical Oncology 2007 update of recommendations for the use of tumor markers in breast cancer. J Clin Oncol 25:1–26
8. Slamon DJ, Clark GM, Wong SG et al (1987) Human breast cancer: correlation of relapse and survival with amplification of the HER-2/neu oncogene. Science 235(4785):177–182
9. Wolff AC, Hammond ME, Schwartz JN et al (2007) American Society of Clinical Oncology/ College of American Pathologists guideline recommendation for human epidermal growth factor receptor 2 testing in breast cancer. Arch Pathol Lab Med 25:118–145
10. Jansen RL, Hupperets PS, Arends JW et al (1998) MIB-1 labelling index is an independent prognostic marker in primary breast cancer. Br J Cancer 78:460–465

11. Sotiriou C, Wirapati P, Loi S et al (2006) Gene expression profiling in breast cancer: understanding the molecular basis of histologic grade to improve prognosis. J Natl Cancer Inst 98(4):262–272
12. Pinder SE, Provenzano E, Earl H, Ellis IO (2007) Laboratory handing and histology reporting of breast specimens from patients who have received neoadjuvant chemotherapy. Histopathology 50:409–417
13. Jeruss JS, Mittendorf EA, Tucker SL et al (2008) Staging of breast cancer in the neoadjuvant setting. Cancer Res 68:6477–6481

Index